# The GP Quiz Book 2

## Further detection and management of physical disease

Alick Munro

RADCLIFFE MEDICAL PRESS

Radcliffe Medical Press Ltd
18 Marcham Road, Abingdon, Oxon OX14 1AA

British Library Cataloguing in Publication Data
A catalogue record for this book is available from the British Library.

ISBN 1 85775 383 6

Typeset by Joshua Associates Ltd, Oxford
Printed and bound by TJ International Ltd, Padstow, Cornwall

# Contents

# Preface

Some of the best clinical teachers I had as a student and junior hospital doctor used to conduct their tutorials and ward rounds as quizzes. Sometimes the answers were unknown even to them, but the format stimulated thought, discussion and library searches. I used to think it unfortunate that only a small minority of the medical textbooks then available had quizzes on the subject matter as an appendix. Using them allows us to rapidly spot important gaps in our knowledge and direct our reading accordingly. Quizzes also help us to maintain interest in the subject.

When the postgraduate education allowance was introduced in 1990, I started producing quizzes from the content of the *British Medical Journal* and the *British Journal of General Practice*. Both of these journals carry peer-reviewed original research and authoritative reviews. Every 3 months, members of our Doctors' Reading Club earn their PGEA by filling out a quiz review based on recent material in these journals. I formulate the questions with a mind to drawing attention to those matters which came as important news to me, or which seem most likely to influence the thoughts of fellow GPs on how best to practise. Members return the quiz reviews for checking and scoring, and then receive them back with model answers to the factual questions and summaries of their answers to the debatable points contained in our newsletter.

The quiz reviews and the material from the newsletter have now been collated by topic for publication, and also to satisfy our members who required this format for ease of reference. This book and its companion volume are limited to the detection and management of physical disease, and because of this have a preponderance of factual questions. Books on psychological, social preventative and management issues will follow.

How might readers use this book? It does not contain a comprehensive account of any topic. Many of the thought-provoking questions have been addressed by summarizing the points made by the authors of original articles and by members of our Doctors' Reading Club, and by adding comments of my own based on additional reading. The answers are perhaps not the last word on these open-ended subjects. However, the book is designed to be a stimulating read, concentrating on those matters that are most likely to affect how GPs work. It is suited to intermittent browsing, and sometimes that is all a GP has time for. However, I myself find it useful to have the text available as an *aide-mémoire* in the consulting room. Students, trainees and practitioners may find that this format helps them to identify and plug important gaps in their knowledge, and to locate recent authoritative evidence for more detailed study.

I hope you will enjoy the book, and I would like to thank the contributors and editing staff at the journals and the members of Doctors' Reading Club whose writings have provided me with so much interesting information.

Dr Alick Munro MRCP MSc
*July 1999*

# ACCIDENTS AND EMERGENCIES

**1** What is appropriate immediate medical treatment for someone who has polymyalgia, headache and failing vision?

*BMJ.* **315**: 549 (letter)

**2** What should be done to prevent microbial keratitis in the eyes of an unconscious patient? (*3 points*)

*BMJ.* **314**: 433–4 (case reports)

**3** A reliable diagnosis of the absence of fracture can be based on symptoms and signs shortly after an injury which has left the patient feeling shaken. (*True/False*)

*BMJ.* **315**:1230 (anecdotes)

**4** What types of injuries involving broken skin are best left unsutured for the first few days?

*BMJ.* **315**:1146–7

**5** A patient has sustained a deep, clean cut at the wrist or ankle.

**a** What investigation will be useful to determine whether a tendon has been severed?

**b** If the diagnosis of a severed tendon at the ankle has been missed, what long-term problems are likely to ensue?

*BMJ.* **315**:1528–9 (case reports and discussion)

**6** What is the value of a skull X-ray in determining the risk of intracranial injury after a child has suffered a head injury?

*BMJ.* **316**:1758 (citation)

**7** How should the arms be placed for a patient in the recovery position?

*BMJ.* **315**:1230 (anecdotes), 1308 (letter)

**8** What condition in addition to drowning appears to justify a particularly long period of cardiopulmonary resuscitation?

*BMJ.* **313**: 92 (correspondence dated 1896)

**9** What procedures should be used to relieve a child who is choking from food in his airway and gasping for breath?

*BMJ.* **308**: 1349–55

**10** What survival rates would you expect for people suffering cardiac arrest:
**a** if treated by members of the public before the ambulance arrived
**b** if first treated by the ambulance crew?

*BMJ.* **309**: 1242 (citation)

**11** What benefits have been demonstrated for interposed abdominal counter-pulsation during cardiopulmonary resuscitation?

*BMJ.* **314**: 1462–5 (review)

**12** What reflex action may a supine patient take to counteract tissue hypoxia in hypovolaemic shock?

*BMJ.* **315**: 707 (anecdote)

**13** A stuporose patient who has been in an accident opens his eyes only to painful stimuli, his speech is incomprehensible, and he brushes your hand away when you pinch his earlobe.
**a** What is his Glasgow coma score?
**b** What other neurological examination techniques are useful for assessing central nervous system (CNS) damage in a subconscious patient?

*BMJ.* **308**: 1620–4

# ANSWERS

1 A massive intravenous dose of steroid, e.g. 500 mg methylprednisolone or 10 mg dexamethasone IV immediately, followed by admission and 80 mg prednisolone daily while observing visual acuity.

2 Keep the eyes closed. Polyacrylamide gel (Geliperm), taping or even lower lid suture may be helpful. Eye care with antibiotic drops and lubricating ointment every few hours should be instituted. Eyes may be examined with fluorescein to detect early keratitis.

3 False.

4 Blast wounds, as these will probably involve contamination or damage to underlying tissues, which are likely to swell during the first week after injury.

5 a Ultrasound.
  b Fixed deformity, awkward gait, calluses and secondary osteoarthritis.

6 Severe intracranial injuries may occur in the absence of skull fracture. Headache, drowsiness and vomiting are more valuable indicators.

7 With the patient lying on his or her side, the overlying leg flexed at the hip and knee, and the hand of the overlying arm under the face, palm downwards. The underlying arm should be behind the patient, palm upwards.

8 Lightning strike.

9 Back blows with the child prone, chest thrusts with the child supine, expired air ventilation, and abdominal thrusts with the child erect (Heimlich manoeuvre), all performed in rotation.

10 a 25%.
   b 8%.

11 Increased coronary and carotid perfusion and increased cardiac output.

12 Yawn.

13 a The Glasgow coma score is derived as follows.

| Eye opening | |
|---|---|
| Spontaneous | 4 |
| To voice | 3 |
| To pain | 2 |
| None | 1 |

| Best verbal response | |
|---|---|
| Orientated | 5 |
| Confused | 4 |
| Inappropriate words | 3 |

| | |
|---|---|
| Incomprehensible | 2 |
| None | 1 |
| Best motor response | |
| Obeys commands | 6 |
| Localizes pain | 5 |
| Withdraws from pain | 4 |
| Flexes to pain | 3 |
| Extends to pain | 2 |
| None | 1 |

So in this case the score is 2+2+5 = 9.

b Pupil size and response to light, examination of the ears and nose for CSF and blood, looking for blood behind the eardrum, sensation (including the perianal area), tendon reflexes and limb movements.

# ALLERGY

## Aetiology

**1** What factors in prenatal or early life experience may predispose to atopy?

*BMJ.* **314**: 987–8 (leading article)

**2** What is the prevalence of allergic disorder:
**a** in the population as a whole
**b** if one parent is affected
**c** if both parents are affected?

*BMJ.* **316**: 686–9 (review)

**3** List several reactions to food ingestion that are not due to allergy.
(*6 or more points*)

*BMJ.* **316**: 1299–302 (review)

**4** Rhinitis.
**a** Which drugs may induce it? (*5 points*)
**b** Which foods may induce it? (*3 points*)
**c** Which allergen is most likely to cause a perennial form of the disorder?

*BMJ.* **316**: 917–20 (review)

**5** How may diesel fumes enhance allergic responses in the airways?

*BMJ.* **316**: 600–3 (review)

**6** A woman feels faint and develops asthma as well as itch and swelling in the vagina 2 min after a vaginal examination. What is likely to have caused the problem?

*BMJ.* **316**: 1442–5 (review)

# Diagnosis and assessment

**1** How would you differentiate a polyp from a turbinate on examination of the nose? (*4 points*)

*BMJ.* **316**: 917–20 (review)

**2** What blood test performed in the first few hours after onset may confirm a diagnosis of acute anaphylaxis?

*BMJ.* **316**: 1442–5 (review)

**3** Interpreting allergy tests.
  **a** A skin-prick test is positive, but there is no clear history of reaction after exposure to this substance in everyday life. What are the possible explanations for this? (*2 points*)
  **b** What are the limitations of skin testing with food allergens? (*2 points*)
  **c** What can one conclude about effective therapy for rhinitis if there are numerous eosinophils in a smear of nasal secretions? (*1 point*)

*BMJ.* **316**: 686–9 (review)

**4** Food allergy. (*True/False*)
  **a** Patients with true allergic responses to foods usually recognize which food(s) cause the problem.
  **b** Symptoms usually appear within minutes.
  **c** The patient usually has other allergic disorders.

*BMJ.* **316**: 1299–302 (review)

**5** Allergy.
  **a** In what common situations might a skin-prick test for allergy be useful? (*12 points*)
  **b** For how long should antihistamines be discontinued before testing?
  **c** What difficulty arises in interpreting patch-contact tests?

*BMJ.* **316**: 535–7 (review)

**6** Which allergens appear to be worth testing for by skin-prick tests in general practice?

*BMJ.* **316**: 1584–7 (review)

**7** **a** A skin test for allergy is positive. What is the approximate likelihood that the patient has or will have allergic symptoms associated with the allergen concerned?

**b** A 2-year-old child has developed angiooedema within an hour of eating at a restaurant. What further information will you seek? (*5 or more points*)

*BMJ.* **312**: 1074–8 (research report)

**8** Venom allergy. (*True/False*)

**a** Patients give reliable answers when asked whether they were stung by a bee or a wasp.

**b** A child with a generalized reaction to a first sting is very likely to suffer a worse reaction to a subsequent sting.

*BMJ.* **316**: 1365–8 (review)

# Management

**1** Apart from using medication, what can patients with hay fever do to prevent their symptoms? (*10 or more points*)

*BMJ.* **314**: 1392–5 (review)

**2** What common aeroallergens exist in the home, and what can be done to reduce exposure to them? (*10 points*)

*BMJ.* **316**: 1075–8 (review)

**3** Toddlers with proven allergy to ingested allergens may become tolerant to an oral challenge after a few years. (*True/False*)

*BMJ.* **316**: 1271–4 (research report)

**4** What is the best position for the head when using:

**a** a nasal spray

**b** nasal drops?

*BMJ.* **316**: 1584–7 (review)

**5** Hay fever.

    **a** What is the best treatment if the nose is completely blocked?

    **b** What treatments are particularly useful if there is severe watery rhinorrhoea?

*BMJ.* **316**: 843–5 (review)

**6** For what conditions is allergen injection immunotherapy in specialist centres currently indicated? (*2 points*)

*BMJ.* **307**: 919–22

**7** How much 1/1000 adrenalin and by what route would you use to treat severe anaphylaxis in a 70 kg man?

*BMJ.* **305**: 183

**8** Treating anaphylaxis. (*True/False*)

    **a** Intravenous adrenalin is safer than intramuscular adrenalin in moderate cases.

    **b** Only one dose of adrenalin should be given.

    **c** Crystalloid is better than colloid as a plasma expander.

    **d** Prophylaxis with steroids should be considered for subsequent exposure to the allergen.

*BMJ.* **311**: 731–3 (review)

**9** A patient is suffering acute anaphylaxis. How can you prevent further current contact with the allergen:

    **a** if it is an insect sting to the leg

    **b** if the patient has ingested it?

*BMJ.* **311**: 1434 (letter)

**10** If a child at risk of anaphylaxis is prescribed syringes of adrenalin for emergency use, who should be shown how to use them?

*BMJ.* **312**: 638 (letter)

# ANSWERS

## Aetiology

1  Being the first born, suffering relatively few infectious illnesses in early life, and avoiding contact with other infants and children. These are factors that cause Th lymphocytes to be expressed as Th2 rather than Th1 lymphocytes, and this predisposes to atopy. Suspicion that fetal undernutrition in the latter stages of pregnancy may predispose to atopy is also under investigation.

2  a  10–20%.
   b  50%.
   c  75%.

3  • Tyramine in cheese or red wine may provoke migraine.
   • Monosodium glutamate may provoke flushing, headache and abdominal symptoms – Chinese restaurant syndrome.
   • Lactase deficiency in young children results in abdominal symptoms and diarrhoea after ingesting milk.
   • Scombroid in rotting oily fish contains histamine and may cause flushing, hypotension and urticaria.
   • Benzoic acid in citrus fruit may cause a perioral flare-up in children.
   • Food additives, particularly preservatives, may cause flare-ups of urticaria, or asthma.

4  a  Beta-blockers, ACE inhibitors, chlorpromazine, oral contraceptives and NSAIDs.
   b  Hot spices, food colourings and preservatives, and alcohol.
   c  House-dust mite.

5  Polyaromatic hydrocarbons in diesel fumes increase the IgE response to common inhaled allergens.

6  An anaphylactic reaction to latex gloves.

## Diagnosis and assessment

1  Polyps are usually pale grey, translucent and mobile, and lack any sensation on gentle probing.

2  Mast cell tryptase, which peaks 1 h after the onset of anaphylaxis.

3  a Exposure may be perennial, so the patient does not notice acute reactions, or the substance presented to the skin when testing may be a cross-reactant and not the allergen to which the patient is exposed in daily life.

   b Food allergens do not reliably give positive results on skin testing. Skin reactions to food allergens include anaphylaxis, so adrenalin should be available when they are tested in this way.

   c Corticosteroids are likely to be effective.

4  a True.

   b True.

   c True.

5  a • To determine whether removing a pet is likely to alleviate an allergy problem.

     • To determine whether there is allergy to house-dust mite that may justify precautions and adaptations.

     • To identify whether food allergens such as milk, eggs, fish, shellfish or nuts may be contributing to a patient's symptoms.

     • To identify sensitivity to mould, insect and plant allergens in those who are occupationally exposed to them.

   b 48 h or 21 days if they have a long half-life.

   c It may be impossible to establish whether a reaction is due to chemical irritation or to cell-mediated allergy.

6  House-dust mite, grass pollen, and dog and cat hair according to the original article.

7  a One in three.

   b • What food and drink was consumed?

     • What were the ingredients?

     • Did the food or drink contain nuts, eggs, milk, pulses, wheat, banana, avocado, fish or sesame?

     • Have similar reactions occurred previously?

     • Does the child have other features of allergy (skin, nose, eyes, airways or gut)?

8  a False.

   b False – subsequent stings may provoke no reaction or a milder reaction.

# Management

1  • Avoid going out when the pollen count is highest. Information on the pollen count is available by telephoning 01705 77 77 220. The pollen count is usually highest in the evening.

   • Avoid car travel in the evening rush-hour in urban areas. Buy a car with an air filter.

   • Avoid picnics, camping and mowing grass.

- Shower and wash hair on returning from trips to the countryside.
- Wear wrap-around sunglasses when outside.
- Bring in washing before the evening.
- Close windows and car windows.
- Avoid tobacco smoke and other irritants such as fresh paint.

2 • *House-dust mite.* Cover the mattress, pillows and duvet with covers that are impermeable to mite allergens. Wash all exposed bedding at 55° C. Replace bedroom carpets with vinyl or wooden flooring. Curtains should be hot washed regularly, and intensive vacuum-cleaning is needed elsewhere with a high-efficiency particulate air filter and double-thickness bags, or use a steam cleaner on carpets to kill mites.
- *Dog and cat hair.* Either get rid of the pet, or keep it out of the way of the allergy sufferer. Remove carpets, or clean them with a high-efficiency particulate air cleaner.
- *Cockroach allergens.* These may be important in schools and high-rise flats.

3 True.

4 a Bend the neck forward.
  b Lie flat on the back with the neck extended over the edge of the couch. Remain in this position for 2 min after application of the drops.

5 a Oral steroid, e.g. 20 mg prednisolone daily for 5 days.
  b A decongestant, e.g. ipratropium bromide.

6 Seasonal allergic rhinitis and bee-sting sensitivity that is unresponsive to medical treatment.

7 0.35–0.55 mL IV.

8 a False – it should only be used in severe cases, as it carries a higher risk of ventricular arrhythmia.
  b False – about 10% of patients require a second bolus after 5 min.
  c False – colloid stays in the circulation for longer.
  d True – however, antihistamines may be useful for this purpose, and some patients carry a loaded syringe of adrenalin.

9 a Apply a tourniquet.
  b Rinse out the mouth and use an emetic.

10 Both the child and his or her parents and other adults who are regularly left in charge of the child.

# ANTIBIOTICS

**1** What rules on antibiotic prescribing should be adopted in order to limit the spread of antibiotic resistance? (*3 or more points*)

*Br J Gen Pract.* **47**: 415–16 (leading article)

**2** What percentage of pneumococcal isolates in England and Wales have been found to show intermediate or full resistance to the following antibiotics?

**a** Penicillin.

**b** Tetracycline.

**c** Erythromycin.

**d** Trimethoprim.

**e** Rifampicin.

**f** Ampicillin.

*BMJ.* **312**: 1454–6 (research report)

**3** Data on children's carriage of penicillin-resistant pneumococci support the following conclusions. (*True/False*)

**a** Using antibiotics other than penicillin for routine infections will reduce the problem.

**b** Most penicillin-resistant pneumococci resist most other oral antibiotics as well.

**c** In the absence of exposure to antibiotics, carriage of penicillin-resistant pneumococci disappears within about 9 months.

**d** In the first few weeks after a course of antimicrobial treatment, penicillin-resistant pneumococci are more likely than not to be present in a child's nose.

*BMJ.* **313**: 387–90 (research report)

**4** List eight antibacterial agents to which methicillin-resistant *Staphylococcus aureus* is likely to be sensitive.

*BMJ.* **307**: 1049–52

BMJ. **304**: 1135

**5** According to guidelines from the British Society for Antimicrobial Chemotherapy, patients with congenital or valvular heart disease should receive antibiotic prophylaxis before the following procedures: (*True/False*)

**a** minor dental procedures

**b** ear, nose and throat (ENT) procedures

**c** urinary catheterization

**d** insertion of an intrauterine contraceptive device (IUCD)

**e** gastroscopy.

*Drug Ther Bull.* **28**: 90–2

**6** Antibiotic prophylaxis before dentistry is recommended for patients with the following conditions: (*True/False*)

**a** hip replacement

**b** Spitz-Holter valve.

*BMJ.* **307**:1993–4

**7** What are the indications that may justify prolonged courses of intravenous antimicrobials? (*5 or more points*)

*BMJ.* **313**: 1541–3 (discussion and report)

**8** List three means by which patients may form a mistaken impression that they are 'sensitive to penicillin'.

*BMJ.* **302**: 1462–3

**9** The authors suggest that patients who give a history of 'penicillin allergy' should be tested by a radioallergosorbent test on venous blood. Those with no IgE antibodies to penicillin can then be given an oral challenge under medical supervision with resuscitation facilities available. In which groups of patients with penicillin allergy might this procedure be justified?

*BMJ.* **302**: 1051–2

**10** The following anti-infectives penetrate tissue well: (*True/False*)

**a** amoxycillin

**b** erythromycin

**c** cotrimoxazole

**d** cephalexin

**e** doxycycline

**f** ciprofloxacin.

*Br J Gen Pract.* **41**: 38

**11** Antibiotics after a dog bite.

**a** What risk factors may justify prophylactic antibiotics? (*8 points*)

**b** What are the two antibiotics of choice for adults?

*BMJ.* **314**: 88–9 (leading article)

**12** Which antibacterial agent commonly used in treatment of urinary tract infections (UTIs) has least effect on the bowel flora?

*Br J Gen Pract.* **42**: 138–9

**13** What particular risk is there in prescribing cotrimoxazole for an elderly patient?

*BMJ.* **306**: 698

**14** What commonly used antibiotic is also useful for treating delayed gastric emptying?

*BMJ.* **307**: 1084

**15** What delayed consequence has been associated with a high rate of erythromycin prescribing for upper respiratory tract infections (URTIs)?

*BMJ.* **313**:890 (citation)

**16** What warning should be given to patients for whom ciprofloxacin is prescribed?

*BMJ.* **309**: 542

**17** What antibiotic has been reported to cause tinnitus?

*BMJ.* **311**: 232

**18** Which antibiotic injection should be available for a GP who wishes to be able to provide emergency treatment for meningococcal septicaemia in a patient with a history of penicillin allergy?

*BMJ.* **304**: 116

# ANSWERS

1 According to the author:
- limit prescribing to conditions which require antibiotic treatment
- rely on local information on likely pathogens and their pattern of resistance
- use an effective antibiotic in an effective dose for as short a course as is likely to be effective.

2 a 3.9%.
  b 5.1%.
  c 8.6%.
  d 18%.
  e 0%.
  f 2.7%.

3 a False.
  b True.
  c True.
  d True.

4 Neomycin, mupirocin, fusidic acid, ciprofloxacin, rifampicin, vancomycin, teicoplanin and chlorhexidine.

5 a True.
  b True.
  c False.
  d False.
  e False.

6 a False.
  b False.

7 Osteomyelitis, septic arthritis, infections complicating AIDS, cystic fibrosis and cancer.

8 • They suffer a skin eruption due to an infection for which penicillin is prescribed.
  • They hear the doctor say 'sensitive to penicillin' when referring to a culture result.
  • They are sensitive to a particular semisynthetic penicillin, not to the penicillin nucleus.

9 Those who may particularly need penicillin treatment, namely:
- patients with cystic fibrosis
- patients with sickle-cell disease
- some chronic bronchitics

- splenectomized patients.

**10** **a** False.

    **b** True.

    **c** True.

    **d** False.

    **e** True.

    **f** True.

A practical application is that penicillins and cephalosporins are not useful for treating UTIs in males, as they do not penetrate the prostate.

**11** **a** Wounds to the hands or feet, or that are more than 8 h old or have undergone primary closure, or which are crush or puncture wounds.

    Patients aged over 50 years or who are female or have alcoholic liver disease or asplenism, or who are immunosuppressed.

    **b** Co-amoxiclav, doxycycline.

**12** Nitrofurantoin.

**13** Folate deficiency leading to pancytopenia.

**14** Erythromycin.

**15** Increased incidence of meningococcal meningitis.

**16** It may cause drowsiness. If affected, do not drive.

**17** Ciprofloxacin.

**18** Chloramphenicol.

# BACK PAIN

**1** What physical observations may help to determine whether a patient complaining of low back pain has a genuine pain? (*7 points*)

*BMJ.* **305**: 7–8

**2** A patient has suffered lumbago for 2 days. What sociodemographic factors and observations on history and physical examination will most affect the prognosis? (*6 points*)

*BMJ.* **308**: 577–80

**3** Is a lumbar spine X-ray required for the following patients? State your point of view and a reason for it.

**a** A 27-year-old nurse who strained her back 2 weeks ago has been resting since then, but her back pain is no better. She has pain on straight-leg raising and a reduced knee jerk on one side.

**b** A 35-year-old man has a history of many years of increasing backache that is worse in the mornings and is relieved by exercise. Lumbar flexion is much reduced but he has no neurological signs.

**c** A 68-year-old man with a 3-month history of increasing backache also has increasing urinary retention and dipstick haematuria. Lumbar movements are normal and he has no neurological signs.

**d** An 80-year-old woman with a kyphosis has had previous episodes of backache. She has been bedridden for 2 days with the latest episode, which came on suddenly while she was walking to the door.

*BMJ.* **313**: 1343 (editorial)

**4** RCGP guidelines on managing back pain include the following precepts. (*True/False*)

**a** 'Let pain be your guide' when deciding how much exercise is appropriate.

**b** Use analgesics on demand.

**c** Spinal manipulation may be considered within 6 weeks of onset of symptoms.

*BMJ.* **313**: 1343 (editorial)

**5** Traction can be recommended for a patient with back pain of mechanical origin and onset 3 days previously. (*True/False*)

*BMJ.* **309**: 1602 (summary of report)

**6** What facilities around the house may make life easier for someone who suffers from chronic back pain? (*3 points*)

*BMJ.* **306**: 901–8

**7** What criteria would you use to select patients with lumbago who might suitably be referred for a programme of fitness training? (*4 or more points*)

*BMJ.* **310**: 151–4 (research report)

**8** Patients with low back pain of mechanical origin would be best served if their GPs provided a service of spinal manipulation. Do you agree with this? State reasons for your point of view. (*3 or more points*)

*BMJ.* **311**: 349–51 (original research)

**9** Patients with a history of several consultations for back pain, but who no longer consult their GPs with this problem, are likely to be free of it. (*True/False*)

*BMJ.* **316**: 356–9 (research report)

**10** In an observer-blind trial of the treatment of chronic backstrain and neckstrain we should expect the following:

**a** the drop-out rate to be higher with medicinal treatment and self-treatment than with treatment by a therapist

**b** the drop-out rate to be exactly the same with sham treatment by a therapist and with active treatment by a therapist

**c** manipulation to be only slightly better than physiotherapy, i.e. massage, exercises and/or radiation.

*BMJ.* **304**: 601–5

**11** Back pain in otherwise healthy physically active men may be due to ischaemia. Do you believe this? State reasons for your point of view. (*2 points*)

*BMJ.* **306**: 1267–8

*BMJ.* **309**: 1267–9 (research report)

12 What useful information on management of back pain has yet to be gained from research that could best be conducted in general practice? (*3 or more points*)

*BMJ.* **312**: 485–9 (review article)

# ANSWERS

1  The following signs suggest malingering or hypochondriacal pain:
   - over-reaction
   - closing the eyes during the examination
   - pain on rotation of the shoulders and pelvis together
   - pain when pressure is applied to the top of the head
   - pain on straight-leg raising but not on bending forward to touch the toe or when sitting up on the couch
   - superficial tenderness not corresponding to the distribution of a nerve
   - loss of power that is regional and jerky, suddenly giving way.

2  - Past history of back pain.
   - The severity of the initial disability.
   - Pain that is worse on standing or on lying down.
   - Awaiting judgement on compensation.
   - Job satisfaction.
   - Being male is associated with delayed return to work.

3  a  There appears to be no good reason for requesting a lumbar spine X-ray for the 27-year-old nurse with a history of backstrain. Exposure to X-rays while of reproductive age is a particular deterrent. If the problem persists, an orthopaedic referral is the preferred option.
   b  The 35-year-old man with a history suggestive of ankylosing spondylitis might require an X-ray for a causal diagnosis, but lymphocyte antigen studies would also be of value.
   c  The man with a history suggestive of prostatic carcinoma needs a urological referral and perhaps a bone scan, rather than an X-ray.
   d  The elderly woman with a history of osteoporotic fracture might require an X-ray to determine whether osteomalacia is contributing to the problem. However, Looser zones are more likely to be found in the pubic rami and long bones than in the lumbar spine. Moving this patient to the radiology department would be a particular problem. Most doctors would not request an X-ray in these circumstances.

4  a  False – mild pain should not contraindicate exercise.
   b  False – the guideline promotes regular dosing.
   c  True.

5  False.

6  Raised bed, toilet and chair, a kneeler chair to maintain lumbar lordosis, and a gripper to extend use of the arm without the patient needing to rise from the bed or chair.

7 Most GPs answering this question agree that mobilization is part of the treatment of any back-pain sufferer whose problem is primarily mechanical or due to ankylosing spondylitis, and who is free of nerve root signs or other physical limitations. Unwillingness to take part in such a programme may be tackled with persuasive discussion, analgesics, muscle relaxants and occasionally with antidepressants. Practical considerations may require that some patients undertake their own mobilization programme rather than attending a physiotherapy department. If so, they will benefit from having suitable exercises demonstrated to them, and from regular follow-up by a GP who takes the trouble to measure their range of pain-free movement and to encourage and congratulate them appropriately.

8 The consensus view in reviews of the subject is that back pain of mechanical origin is reduced by spinal manipulation, which is best undertaken between 2 and 30 days after onset. However, the benefit may be only temporary. The treatment is safe provided that it is restricted to those who are free of fracture, tumour, inflammatory joint disease or advanced osteoporosis and, in the case of cervical manipulation, also free from brainstem ischaemia, and any condition such as rheumatoid arthritis or Down's syndrome causing atlanto-axial instability.

GPs seem to be well placed to provide this service, as they are accessible and they can employ a full range of other pharmacological and physical treatments for pain. The majority of GPs who expressed an opinion agreed with this view. They mentioned that the service could reduce time lost from work, the expense of visiting private chiropractors, and pressure on hospital physiotherapy and out-patient departments. Revision of the GP contract may encourage GPs to extend their repertoire to include this type of service, which could then be provided to patients of neighbouring practices.

Those who disagreed with the suggestion were concerned that undertrained GPs offering the service in a hurry might bring it into disrepute, that the intervention has not yet been adequately evaluated, and that it encourages patients to adopt the sick role for what is usually a self-limiting problem.

9 False – only 25% of patients who had consulted their GPs with back pain in this study were free of the problem at follow-up 12 months later.

10 a True.

b False.

c True.

11 Back pain has been associated with cardiovascular risk factors, particularly smoking, and with atherosclerotic lumbar arteries in cadavers. In farmers aged 30–49 years, back pain was found to be significantly ($p=0.04$) associated with future coronary heart disease after adjusting for smoking, age, body mass index and social status. However, if back pain is due to ischaemia, it is strange that a similar association was not found in patients over the age of 50 years, unless the back pain in older men is more commonly due to degenerative disease rather than to mechanical injuries. It is possible that ischaemia might delay healing of mechanical damage. Alternatively, lack of regular exercise might be a common determinant of both conditions, or low

back pain may cause lack of exercise, which in turn causes ischaemic heart disease. Despite these uncertainties, the association does appear to be worth mentioning to middle-aged smokers who suffer back pain.

12  GPs suggested that the following areas of uncertainty might usefully be addressed by research in general practice.

- How specific and predictive are the risk features in the history (e.g. unremitting night pain) and the physical signs that appear to justify referral (e.g. reduced straight-leg raising, decreased tendon jerks, reduced power or sensation) in patients in different age groups?
- Which patients are helped by manipulation?
- Does early mobilization influence recovery if there is sciatica as well as lumbago?
- Which patients comply with advice on early mobilization?
- Does it help to provide an information booklet on exercise?
- If patients benefit from manipulation, does it help to show their relatives how to perform this procedure?
- Which patients benefit from cognitive therapy to tackle the somatization factor?

Other areas of ignorance require a joint approach with specialist departments. In this category GPs suggested the following.

- What is the diagnostic yield of scanning techniques in different subgroups of patients?
- Which patients benefit from epidural injection, which from surgery, and which from chemonucleolysis?

# BREAST CONDITIONS

## Aetiology

**1** Early detection of breast cancer. (*True/False*)

  **a** Women whose mothers developed breast cancer when they were relatively young are at more risk than those whose mothers developed breast cancer in later life.

  **b** Early menarche is a risk factor for breast cancer.

  **c** A history of numerous pregnancies is a risk factor for breast cancer.

  **d** Women at very high risk of breast cancer and aged under 50 years should have mammograms every 3 years.

  *BMJ.* **308**: 183–7

**2** If one in 12 women develop breast cancer, what proportion of women with a first-degree relative with breast cancer develop it? (*based on a study in Utah – 1 point*)

  *BMJ.* **307**: 1016

**3** Breast cancer is familial, but what features of the proband case(s) are associated with particular risk in relatives? (*3 points*)

  *BMJ.* **315**:1244 (citations)

**4** What relative risk of breast cancer does a woman over 55 years of age incur if she has taken HRT for more than 5 years?

  *BMJ.* **310**: 1684

# Diagnosis

**1** Self-examination.

    **a** What proportion of women know how and why to examine their breasts?

    **b** What proportion do so monthly?

    *BMJ.* **316**: 1463 (letter)

**2** What proportion of women who detected a breast lump delayed revealing it for 6 months or longer in this study?

    *BMJ.* **316**: 1744 (letter)

**3** What information or suggestions would you put to a woman aged 50–64 years who has declined to attend for mammography? (*5 or more points*)

    *BMJ.* **309**: 168–74

**4** Breast conditions. *(15 points)*

    **a** How would you position a woman to palpate her breasts?

    **b** How would you detect deep fixation of a breast lump?

    **c** How might you differentiate a breast cyst from a breast tumour from the history?

    **d** What age group of women may benefit from an ultrasound examination of the breast if a breast lump is detected on examination?

    **e** What is the disadvantage of a GP performing a needle biopsy?

    **f** What information would you seek if a woman complains of a nipple discharge:

    **g** What is the positive predictive value of the following findings for a breast carcinoma:

      i a solitary lump on clinical examination

      ii a solitary tumour on mammography

      iii malignant cells on cytology from a needle biopsy of a breast tumour?

    *BMJ.* **309**: 722–6

**5** When aspirating a breast cyst, why should the fluid be sent for electrolyte assay?

    *BMJ.* **314**: 925–8 (research report)

**6** Once testing is available for the BRCA1 gene which predisposes to breast and ovarian cancer:

**a** who should be tested

**b** what are the implications of a positive result for risk of breast and ovarian cancer

**c** what are the implications of a positive result for further screening

**d** what are the implications of a positive result for further treatment?

*BMJ.* **313**: 572 (leading article)

**7** The following emotional or behavioural responses to a diagnosis of breast cancer may be associated with a good prognosis: (*True/False*)

**a** desire to live an active life and fight the problem

**b** denial of the problem

**c** anxiety

**d** fatalism.

*BMJ.* **302**: 1219–21

# Treatment

**1** For a woman with mild to moderate mastalgia, which preventative treatment would you suggest first? If it failed, which treatment would you suggest second, and which would you suggest third?

*BMJ.* **304**: 194

**2** Mastalgia. (*6 points*)

**a** If danazol is required for cyclical mastalgia, what is the introductory dose?

**b** What side-effects are common with danazol?

**c,** What treatments are available for non-cyclical breast pain?

*BMJ.* **30**: 866–8

**3** How would you drain a breast abscess? (*3 points*)

*BMJ.* **309**:946–9

**4** In descending order of importance, list the benefits that a woman with excessively large breasts may expect as a result of breast reduction surgery. (*4 points*)

*BMJ.* **33**: 454–7 (research report)

**5**    How would you manage eczema confined to the nipple area in a middle-aged woman?

*BMJ.* **309**: 722–6

**6**    Patients referred for treatment of breast cancer are likely to have the disease staged and treated in accordance with a protocol on optimal management agreed by most breast surgeons. (*True/False*)

*BMJ.* **307**: 168–70

**7**    Breast cancer patients can benefit from psychological support. How and where can this best be provided?

*BMJ.* **312**: 813–16 (research report)

**8**    Which problems are likely to cause distress to the following groups of breast cancer patients? (*7 points*)

   **a** Radiotherapy patients.

   **b** Mastectomy patients.

*Br J Gen Pract.* **44**: 370–1

**9**    Chemotherapy for breast cancer. (*True/False*)

   **a** Visual disturbance related to tamoxifen treatment justifies withdrawal of the drug.

   **b** Dexamethasone is useful in the treatment of vomiting related to cytotoxic chemotherapy.

   **c** Oestrogen cream is the first line of treatment for vaginal dryness due to chemotherapy.

*BMJ.* **309**: 1363–6 (review)

**10**    Tamoxifen treatment for breast cancer should be limited to post-menopausal women and those with evidence of metastases. (*True/False*)

*BMJ.* **316**: 1557 (news item)

**11**    What benefits and what drawbacks have been shown for 20 mg tamoxifen daily over 4 years when used to prevent breast cancer in women at high risk? (*4 points*)

*BMJ.* **316**: 1187 (news item)

**12** What symptomatic side-effects have been found in higher prevalence among women using adjuvant tamoxifen than in controls? (*3 points*)

*BMJ.* **313**:1484 (letter)

**13** It is advantageous to continue to prescribe tamoxifen for more than 5 years after a breast tumour has been excised. (*True/False*)

*BMJ.* **312**: 389–90 (leader)

**14** In a follow-up check after mastectomy for breast cancer, what symptom check-list, examination and investigations would seem to be appropriate? (*5 or more points*)

*BMJ.* **313**: 664–7 (research report)

*BMJ.* **310**: 685–6

**15** What treatments are available for lymphoedema of the arm? (*5 points*)

*BMJ.* **309**:1222–5 (review)

# ANSWERS

## Aetiology

1  a  True.
   b  True.
   c  False.
   d  False.

2  One in five.

3  Onset at an early age, bilateral cancer, the presence of oncogenes, and multiple relatives affected.

4  1.71.

## Diagnosis

1  a  90–99%.
   b  15–40%.

2  48 of 170, including many elderly women and two lactating women.

3  Women who have ignored their invitation to attend for mammography may usefully be asked why they have declined to do so. Some are likely to be unconcerned about the risk of breast cancer and need reminding that one in 12 women will develop the disease.

   Some women may be too busy to attend, and these should be encouraged to seek an alternative appointment at a convenient time. Some may have heard that the test is painful or that there are long queues or delays at the X-ray department. If these concerns are well founded, the matter should be resolved. Otherwise, the woman should be reassured that mammography is no more painful than, for example, a venepuncture or a cervical smear. Some may think that the screening would make no difference, and these women may be told that an earlier diagnosis leads to less radical treatment and a better prognosis.

   Some women may dread the disease so much that they prefer to live in ignorance. They may benefit from reassurance that the diagnosis rate is only about 6 per 1000 women screened, and that most probably they will have all their fears allayed.

   Some women may feel that manual examination alone is adequate, and may be told that although self-examination is a very useful technique, there are some tumours that only show up on X-ray.

Some women may be fatalistic. For these, one doctor suggested exerting moral pressure along the lines of 'Do your family think you should attend?' or 'What would your family wish for you?'

4   a  She should be supine with her arms behind her head.

    b  The patient should press her hands on her hips.

    c  A breast cyst may appear quickly and thus have been absent when the woman previously examined her breasts a few weeks ago, whereas a tumour will enlarge slowly.

    d  Premenopausal women, as ultrasound is useful for differentiating tumours from cysts and benign lesions, which have better demarcated edges than do malignant tumours.

    e  Subsequent bruising may make further clinical examination difficult.

    f  What colour is the discharge? Does it contain blood? Is it from one or more ducts? Is it from one breast or from both?

    g   i  95%.

      ii  95%.

     iii  99.8%.

5  If the ratio of potassium to sodium is more than 1.5, the cyst is of type 1, associated with a 4-fold increased risk of future breast cancer, whereas if it is of type 2, with a potassium/sodium ratio of less than 1.5, there is considerably less risk.

6   a  Women with two blood relatives who have developed either breast cancer before the age of 50 years or ovarian cancer before the age of 60 years (suggestion from one expert). A lower threshold for testing is appropriate for Ashkenazi Jews, as they have a higher incidence of the gene.

    b  A 50% risk of breast cancer by the age of 50 years, an 85% risk by the age of 70 years and a 44–63% risk of ovarian cancer.

    c  Consider annual mammograms from the age of 35 years.

    d  Consider prophylactic tamoxifen if post-menopausal.
Consider oophorectomy

7   a  True.

    b  True.

    c  False.

    d  False.

# Treatment

1  The author suggests evening primrose oil, then danazol, and then bromocriptine.

2  a  200–300 mg daily, and reduce to 100 mg daily after 1 month if the patient's pain is relieved.

   b  Acne, hirsutism, weight gain and headache.

   c  A firm supporting bra, NSAIDs, injection of local anaesthetic and steroid treatment.

3  Apply EMLA cream. wait for 1 h, and then aspirate through a 19-gauge needle, reinserted repeatedly if necessary.

4  Less pain, improved physical function, more energy and vitality, better social function, better mental health, and increased participation in physical and mental activity.

5  Refer the patient for surgical care.

6  False – there is enormous variation in practice.

7  The results of this study suggest that such care is best provided by a specialist breast care nurse based at the surgical unit, who is aware of the surgical procedures and facilities for aftercare.

8  a  Depression, weakness, fatigue and sickness.

   b  Problems with the prosthesis, self-image affected by loss of the breast, and residual problems with the arm.

9  a  True.

   b  True.

   c  False – a non-hormonal cream (e.g. Replens) should be tried first.

10  False – the results of a recent trial indicate its use for breast cancer irrespective of age, lymphatic spread or prior chemotherapy.

11  The following benefits have been shown:
   • a halving of the incidence of recurrent breast cancer; in this large-scale study there were 85 cases of breast cancer in the treated group, compared to 154 cases in the women on placebo
   • a lower incidence of fracture; in this study there were 47 fractures of hip, wrist or spine in the treated group, compared to 71 such fractures in the placebo group
   • a halving of the risk of ischaemic heart disease.
   The following drawbacks have been shown:
   • endometrial cancer is more common; there were 33 cases of endometrial carcinoma in the treated group, compared to 14 cases in the placebo group
   • venous thrombosis is more common; there were 17 cases of pulmonary embolus and 30 cases of deep vein thrombosis (DVT) in the treated group, compared to 6 and 9 cases, respectively, in the placebo group.

12  Hot flushes (47% vs. 16%), weight gain (44% vs. 18%) and vaginal discharge (28% vs. 3%).

13  False – trials conducted by the National Cancer Institute in America and a meta-

analysis by the Food and Drug Administration and the results of the Scottish Tamoxifen Trial concluded that continuation of tamoxifen after 5 years conferred no advantage, and the FDA meta-analysis concluded that tamoxifen may be associated with an increased incidence of new tumours in the contralateral breast.

14 Many doctors now doubt the value of frequent follow-up in the clinic or the surgery after treatment for breast cancer. Treatable recurrences in the breasts are most likely to be detected by regular self-examination or regular mammography. If other recurrences are to come to light earlier, it might be better to provide patients with a list of features to bring to medical attention quickly. However, the presentations of regional and metastatic disease are very varied, so the list would be a long and alarming one, including pain at the scar, nodules under the skin, shortness of breath, persistent cough, bone or joint pain, fatigue, malaise, abdominal discomfort, jaundice, headache, vomiting and abnormal bleeding.

This symptom check-list might be better discussed at regular meetings with a GP or practice nurse, and followed by examination of the breasts and the axillary and supraclavicular nodes and the liver edge. Only one doctor responding to this question suggested routine checks of the full blood count, chest X-ray and liver function tests.

15 Oral bioflavonoid oxerutins or coumarins, bandaging the arm, an elastic compression sleeve which is best individually measured for the patient, and a multiple-chamber Flowtron pump used for 2 h per day.

# CARDIOLOGY

## Resuscitation

**1** In cardiopulmonary resuscitation:

   **a** how should the patient's head be held in order to keep the airway open? (*2 points*)

   **b** what else should the resuscitator do with his or her hands while breathing into the patient's mouth? (*1 point*)

   **c** when pressing on the lower sternum, for how long should the pressure be maintained? (*1 point*)

   **d** under what circumstances is an initial precordial thump likely to be helpful? (*1 point*)

   **e** what drug treatment is indicated for a pulseless, apnoeic patient who collapsed within the previous 2 min, in the absence of an ECG or defibrillator? (*1 point*)

*BMJ.* **306**: 1587–93

**2** Why is an inability to read ECGs no bar to using a defibrillator? (*1 point*)

*Br J Gen Pract.* **43**: 95

**3** The British Heart Foundation guidelines for the management of patients with myocardial infarction recommend that GPs should have available certain drugs. Compare your list of suggestions with theirs. (*11 points*)

*BMJ.* **308**: 767–71

**4** Should you in your circumstances have the following items in your car when on call:

   **a** an ECG machine

**b** a thrombolytic drug?

BMJ. **305**: 445–8, 548–53, 846–7, 1014–15

# Chest pain and ischaemia

**1** From the findings cited in this report, what proportion of patients with symptoms suggestive of angina report them to their GPs? (*1 point*)

BMJ. **314**: 257–60 (survey report)

**2** Stable angina pectoris. (*True/False*)

**a** Symptom severity and frequency are good measures of the severity of anatomical damage.

**b** Coronary angioplasty has been shown to improve survival.

Br J Gen Pract. **45**: 11–13 (research report)

**3** Coronary artery balloon angioplasty. (*True/False*)

**a** It has an immediate success rate in excess of 90%.

**b** Restenosis within 6 months occurs in less than 20% of cases.

BMJ. **309**: 579–82

**4** From the results of the Grampian region early anistreplase trial, what increase in mortality is associated with each hour of delay in giving thrombolytic treatment to sufferers of acute myocardial infarction after 2 h have elapsed since the onset of chest pain:

**a** at 30 days after the infarct

**b** at 30 months after the infarct?

BMJ. **312**: 212–16 (research report)

**5** Cardiac chest pain may be indicated by the patient either placing the flat of the hand on the chest, or placing the clenched fist on the middle of the chest, or both hands flat on the middle of the chest and drawn outwards.

**a** What is the predictive value for cardiac pain if these responses occur after a request to 'Show me where your pain is and tell me what it feels like' in the setting of a coronary-care unit? (*2 points*)

**b** What would be the effect on the findings if such a study was to be repeated in a setting where less of the observed chest pain is cardiac in origin? (*2 points*)

*BMJ.* **311**: 1660–1 (research report)

**6** A middle-aged woman suffers tight anterior chest pain brought on by strenuous aerobic exercise, but has a negative exercise cardiography test. She is very unlikely to have ischaemic heart disease. (*True/False*)

*BMJ.* **309**: 555–6

**7** The following drugs are likely to affect the interpretation of a treadmill stress test: (*True/False*)

**a** allopurinol

**b** digoxin

**c** antidepressants.

*BMJ.* **305**:808–9

**8** What treatment other than vasodilators, beta-blockers and aspirin is of proven efficacy in unstable crescendo angina? (*1 point*)

*BMJ.* **306**: 871

**9** In the absence of specific contraindications, what are your drugs of first, second and third choice for long-term control of angina? Give reasons for your point of view.

*BMJ.* **312**: 827–30 (guideline)

## Cardiac hypertrophy and heart failure

**1** In what clinical situations encountered by GPs is direct-access echocardiography most likely to be useful? (*3 or more points*)

*BMJ.* **310**: 611–12, 634–6

**2** If the ECG is normal, an echocardiogram is extremely unlikely to reveal left ventricular systolic dysfunction. (*True/False*)

*BMJ.* **312**: 222 (research report)

**3** Left ventricular hypertrophy: (*True/False*)

**a** is a risk factor for myocardial infarction in normotensive subjects

**b** is found in nearly 10% of hypertensives

**c** is as important a predictor of ischaemic heart disease as is multivessel disease

**d** is best detected by electrocardiography

**e** may develop as a result of repeated ischaemia

**f** justifies intensive investigation of other coronary risk factors

**g** reducing it has been shown to prolong life.

*BMJ.* **311**: 273–4

---

**4** What simple functional test correlates well with peak oxygen uptake and long-term survival in heart failure?

*BMJ.* **313**:890 (citation)

---

**5** In treating heart failure: (*True/False*)

**a** a reduced heart rate is associated with lower mortality

**b** beta-blockers reduce mortality

**c** ACE inhibitors reduce heart rate

**d** amlodipine increases heart rate

**e** amiodarone reduces heart rate.

*BMJ.* **316**: 567–8 (leading article)

---

**6** In the treatment of heart failure: (*True/False*)

**a** there is no point in adding a thiazide if a loop diuretic is not sufficient

**b** diuretics should be stopped for 2 days before introducing an ACE inhibitor

**c** cough in a patient with heart failure treated with an ACE inhibitor is most probably due to the ACE inhibitor

**d** quinine increases the risk of digoxin toxicity

**e** low-dose aspirin is contraindicated.

*BMJ.* **303**: 1546

*BMJ.* **308**: 321–8

---

**7** A patient with chronic congestive cardiac failure is breathless at rest despite maximal treatment with diuretics and ACE inhibitors. What other treatment may palliate his condition? (*1 point*)

*BMJ.* **308**: 717

---

**8** What is the lowest dose of the following ACE inhibitors that has been shown to reduce mortality in patients with congestive cardiac failure? (*4 points*)

**a** Captopril.

**b** Enalapril.

**c** Lisinopril.

**d** Ramipril.

*BMJ.* **310**: 973–4

# Arrhythmia

**1** What is the prevalence of atrial fibrillation in people:

**a** in their fifties

**b** in their eighties?

*BMJ.* **311**: 1361–3 (review)

**2** Atrial fibrillation.

**a** Which is the best ECG lead on which to see fibrillation waves?

**b** What conditions need to be considered as possible contraindications before using anti-arrhythmic agents or defibrillation in a patient with atrial fibrillation?

*BMJ.* **311**:1495–8 (review)

**3** **a** What do you consider to be the most cost-effective way of identifying the cardiac rhythm during periods of palpitations which an ambulant patient notes on average twice a week?

*BMJ.* **311**:1562–5 (review)

**4** What benefit might there be in recording an echocardiogram before deciding whether a patient with atrial fibrillation should undergo cardioversion?

*BMJ.* **311**:1562–5 (review)

**5** What is the treatment of choice for atrial fibrillation in the following circumstances?

**a** It is an occasional mild problem.

**b** To control ventricular rate in a patient who also experiences recurrent anxiety attacks.

**c** The patient has left ventricular failure.

**d** The patient is hypertensive.

*BMJ.* **311**: 1631–4 (review)

**6** Which patients with atrial fibrillation should be referred to a cardiologist? (*8 points*)

BMJ. **312**: 175–8 (review)

**7** Anticoagulation at the time of cardioversion of a patient with atrial fibrillation.
   **a** Which patients require it?
   **b** For how long before cardioversion do they require it?
   **c** For how long after cardioversion do they require it?

BMJ. **312**: 112–15 (review)

**8** Roughly how many patients with atrial fibrillation in each of the following categories would need to be treated with warfarin for 1 year in order to prevent one death, stroke, systemic embolus or transient ischaemic attack?
   **a** Aged over 75 years with one or more of hypertension, diabetes, or previous stroke or transient ischaemic attack.
   **b** Aged 65–75 years with one or more of hypertension, diabetes, or previous stroke or transient ischaemic attack.
   **c** Aged under 65 years with one or more of hypertension, diabetes, or previous stroke or transient ischaemic attack.

Br J Gen Pract. **45**: 503 (letter)

**9** Atrial fibrillation. (*True/False*)
   **a** The risk of thromboembolic disease is particularly high if mitral stenosis is the underlying cause.
   **b** The occurrence of atrial fibrillation during an alcoholic binge is a sign of a diseased heart.
   **c** Strokes related to atrial fibrillation have a more benign prognosis than other strokes.
   **d** Patients with paroxysmal atrial fibrillation are at as much risk of stroke as those with chronic atrial fibrillation.

BMJ. **311**: 1425–8 (review)

BMJ. **312**: 45–9 (review)

BMJ. **304**: 1394

**10** Patients with non-rheumatic atrial fibrillation. (*True/False*)
   **a** They have a risk of stroke averaging 5% per annum.
   **b** Stroke in these patients carries a lower mortality than in patients in sinus rhythm.

c The risk of thromboembolic stroke in these patients can be reduced by about 40% by low-intensity treatment with anticoagulants.

d The majority of elderly patients with non-rheumatic atrial fibrillation have contraindications to the use of anticoagulants.

e The risk of stroke in non-rheumatic atrial fibrillation can be reduced by about 25% with aspirin treatment.

*BMJ.* **305**: 1445–6, 1457–9

*BMJ.* **306**: 207

**11** Only a certain proportion of patients with atrial fibrillation for whom anti-coagulants are indicated are receiving them. How might a GP screen his or her practice population to identify those patients who may benefit from anti-coagulants?

*BMJ.* **307**: 1045

**12** The following are absolute or relative contraindications to warfarin treatment for patients in atrial fibrillation. What criteria would you use as cut-off points in this situation?

a Risk of gastrointestinal blood loss.

b Risk of haematuria.

c Alcoholism.

d Using NSAIDs.

e Risk of falls.

f Inability to use treatment reliably.

g Anaemia.

h Coagulation disorder.

i Low platelet count.

j Renal failure.

k Uncontrolled hypertension.

(*13 points*)

*BMJ.* **314**: 1529–30 (survey report)

**13** Anticoagulation for atrial fibrillation.

a What appears to be the optimal INR?

b What reduction in stroke rate per year has been demonstrated using this treatment?

*BMJ.* **314**: 1563–4

**14** What features in the history might suggest that a patient aged over 60 years with atrial fibrillation would derive particular benefit from anticoagulation? (*6 points*)

*BMJ*. **314**: 978–9

**15** Digoxin toxicity. (*True/False*)

**a** A serum digoxin result in the recommended range rules out the possibility of digoxin toxicity.

**b** Digoxin toxicity is more of a risk if the patient is hyperthyroid.

**c** It is more of a risk if the patient is hyperkalaemic.

*BMJ*. **305**: 1149–52

**16** Amiodarone pulmonary toxicity.

**a** With what symptoms may it present?

**b** What are the typical X-ray appearances?

**c** How might one monitor for it?

*BMJ*. **314**: 619–20 (leading article)

# Miscellaneous

**1** Cardiac treatments. (*True/False*)

**a** Digoxin is only useful in the treatment of chronic heart failure if there is atrial fibrillation.

**b** Beta-blockers are of proven benefit in treating heart failure due to idiopathic dilated cardiomyopathy.

**c** Amiodarone is the only commonly used anti-arrhythmic that does not depress cardiac contractility.

**d** Implantable cardioverter defibrillators can be inserted as simply as pacemakers.

*BMJ*. **309**: 1631–4 (review)

**2** The following ECG findings are significant predictors of a cardiac cause of death: (*True/False*)

**a** more than 100 ventricular ectopics during a day or night

**b** R-on-T phenomena

**c** more than 100 supraventricular ectopic beats during a day or night

**d** supraventricular tachycardia

**e** atrial fibrillation

**f** sinoatrial pauses lasting more than 1.5 s during the day

**g** elevation/depression of the ST segment 80 ms after the J-point in lead 1.

*BMJ.* **304**: 356–9

*BMJ.* **309**: 1263–6 (research report)

**3** QT dispersion on an ECG is highly predictive of cardiovascular death in diabetics and others, even when free of cardiovascular symptoms. What extraordinary precautions might be justified in those with abnormal values?

*BMJ.* **316**: 745–6 (research report)

**4** Why may the ECG be of interest in a very underweight patient with no signs of thyroid disease?

*BMJ.* **304**: 1285

**5** A teenage boy whose father died suddenly in his thirties while engaging in strenuous exercise complains of dyspnoea and fleeting chest pains on exercise. The boy denies morbid anxiety about his father's death. What diagnoses should be entertained, what clinical observations made, and what investigations conducted?

*BMJ.* **306**: 409–10

**6** What treatments are available to patients with hypertrophic obstructive cardiomyopathy who are subject to ventricular arrhythmia?

*BMJ.* **309**: 1277–9 (case reports)

**7** A patient has occasional fleeting chest pains and feels unusually tired on exercise. He has a midsystolic click and a late systolic apical murmur. What is the probable diagnosis and what complications may arise?

*BMJ.* **306**: 943–4

# Heart attack

**1** Cardiac arrests outside hospital.

    **a** What popular misconception leads to delay in calling for appropriate help after the onset of acute coronary occlusion?

    **b** What is the standard intended for the interval before arrival of a paramedic with a defibrillator?

*BMJ.* **316**: 1031–2 (leading article)

**2** What advice should be given to receptionists on how to handle calls from the relatives of middle-aged patients with recent onset of chest pain that may be of cardiac origin?

*BMJ.* **304**: 1058

*Br J Gen Pract.* **42**: 145–7

**3** A middle-aged patient with no previous severe illness or recent contact with the surgery telephones at lunchtime while you are doing some paperwork to tell you he has noted moderately severe 'tight' chest pain increasing over the past 3 h, and he feels unable to come to the surgery. He lives 5 minutes' drive away and 15 minutes from the hospital. Do you call an emergency ambulance and ring the medical registrar to tell him that the patient will be coming, or do you offer to visit? Give reasons for your answer.

*BMJ.* **302**: 504–5

**4** What is the significance of proteinuria as a new finding in a patient who has developed chest pain in the past few hours?

*BMJ.* **302**: 53

**5** In the acute care of an elderly patient who has started to experience crushing chest pain within the past hour: (*True/False*)

    **a** transfer to hospital is more important than treatment of pain, arrhythmia and the thrombotic state

    **b** adrenalin is more likely to be needed than atropine

    **c** bundle branch block on the ECG justifies thrombolytic therapy.

*Br J Gen Pract.* **42**: 525–8

**6** What drugs are effective in treating an intermittent platelet plug as opposed to an established thrombus?

*BMJ.* **307**: 1146

**7** It is important that aspirin be given promptly after the onset of a myocardial infarction. (*True/False*)

*Br J Gen Pract.* **45**: 395–6, 504

**8** By what route should analgesia be administered to the victim of a heart attack?

*BMJ.* **308**: 734–5

*BMJ.* **311**: 1719

**9** In treating ischaemic heart disease: (*True/False*)

  **a** delaying the administration of thrombolysis by 1 h in the first 6 h after an infarction increases 35-day mortality by about 2%

  **b** patients with left ventricular dysfunction after a myocardial infarct derive significant benefit from ACE inhibitors, provided that they are not rendered hypotensive

  **c** calcium antagonists have been shown to reduce the risk of reinfarction

  **d** heparin is the treatment of choice for a patient with unstable angina.

*BMJ.* **309**: 1343–50 (review)

**10** In this study of anistreplase for thrombolysis in myocardial infarction in general practice:

  **a** what proportion of GPs who agreed to use anistreplase actually used it during an 18-month period?

  **b** what proportion of patients with myocardial infarction attended by GPs who agreed to use anistreplase actually received that drug?

*Br J Gen Pract.* **310**: 175–9

**11** When you send a patient with a coronary to hospital you can be fairly sure that he or she will receive a thrombolytic as soon as the diagnosis is confirmed. (*True/False*)

*BMJ.* **316**: 274 (survey report)

**12** What percentage of patients admitted to hospital after GP referral with acute myocardial infarction would you expect to have received the following prior to admission?

**a** An intravenous opiate.

**b** Aspirin.

*BMJ.* **316**: 353 (survey report)

**13** One drug and one class of drug are of proven efficacy in the secondary prevention of myocardial infarction. What are they?

*BMJ.* **302**: 91–2

**14** What types of cardiac patients may benefit most from an exercise rehabilitation programme?

*BMJ.* **306**: 731–2

**15** Between 1978 and 1989, by what percentage did coronary mortality among British men aged 30–65 years decline?

*BMJ.* **303**: 701–4

# ANSWERS

## Resuscitation

1    a   Hold the forehead back, and use your fingers to push the patient's chin forward.

      b   Pinch the patient's nose.

      c   60–100 compressions/min. Press for half the duration of each compression.

      d   If the arrest was seen to happen within the previous 2 min.

      e   Probably none, but 1 mg of adrenaline IV every 2–3 min or 3 mg per endotracheal tube every 2–3 min may enhance the efficacy of basic life support.

2    The latest defibrillators are automated to read the ECG and signal when a shock is appropriate.

3    The British Heart Foundation suggestions for your black bag include oxygen, adrenalin, atropine, aspirin, nitrate, frusemide, lignocaine, naloxone, diamorphine, anti-emetic (e.g. metoclopramide) and possibly an injectable beta-blocker.

4    The suggestion of keeping an ECG machine in the car to speed up diagnosis of coronaries did not appeal to most doctors answering this question, who pointed out that patients living in cities have speedy access to paramedics in fully equipped ambulances. ECG machines in GPs' cars are at risk of being stolen, maintaining the batteries can be difficult if the machine is only used occasionally, and finding a mains point in the patient's house may cause delay. Many doctors pointed out that the ECG changes of a myocardial infarct may not develop in the first hour. Several GPs admitted that their knowledge of ECG interpretation was limited.

     However, members who had ECG machines at their surgeries said that they would call for them on their way to a home visit if a relevant diagnosis was in doubt, and several members who work in rural areas are seriously considering investing in an ECG defibrillator and drugs for emergency coronary care.

     Without an ECG machine, the indications for using a thrombolytic drug cannot be satisfied. Of the thrombolytic drugs that are available, streptokinase is reasonably priced and has a satisfactory storage life (3 years), but requires a slow intravenous infusion. In view of the risk that it will provoke production of antibodies, it is best given only once in a patient's lifetime. Financial support would be required before GPs could be expected to carry a stock of the alternative thrombolytics. Several members therefore commented that they would restrict their coronary care to providing pain relief, aspirin and a rapid-onset preparation of glyceryl trinitrate.

     In the *British Journal of General Practice* (42: 525–8), a cardiologist from Aberdeen makes a good case for coronary patients being stabilized at home before being transported to the coronary care unit. Paramedics in the ambulance service may be in the best position to provide this care, but in London at least they are only provided with ECG machines capable of recording three leads. They do not feel confident to diagnose a myocardial infarct and are provided only with aspirin, atropine, lignocaine, adrenalin, oxygen and Entonox as treatments. Only about two in three emergency ambulances in London are equipped with defibrillators and a trained crew. Until training and provision of paramedics improve, GPs still have a role to play in emergency coronary care, even in cities.

# Chest pain and ischaemia

1    Less than 50%.

2    a  False.

      b  True.

3    a  True.

      b  False – 25–50% of cases restenose within 6 months.

4    a  21 in 1000.

      b  69 in 1000.

5    a  In a coronary-care unit the positive predictive value is 77% and the negative predictive value is 53%.

      b  If the study is repeated in a setting where less of the chest pain is cardiac in origin, the positive predictive value will be lower and the negative predictive value will be higher. However, the sensitivity and specificity will remain unchanged.

6    False – a sensitivity of only 76% is quoted for exercise ECGs in women.

7    a  True.

      b  True.

      c  True.

8    Heparin.

9    The guideline suggests that the first choice is a beta-blocker, as it has been shown to reduce mortality after myocardial infarction and the incidence of vascular events in hypertension. Patients who are intolerant of a beta-blocker should be treated with verapamil, as this drug reduces the rate of major adverse events after myocardial infarction. Nitrates and nicorandil are also effective. Any combinations of the above are useful, with the following cautions and exceptions.

   • Beta-blockers plus verapamil may produce dangerous cardiac failure, so a dihydropyridine calcium antagonist is a better choice of calcium antagonist to use in combination with a beta-blocker.

   • Isosorbide mononitrate rather than isosorbide dinitrate should be used in combination with beta-blockers. Neither form of isosorbide has been demonstrated to be of benefit in combination with calcium channel blockers.

There is no evidence that adding a third drug confers further benefit.

# Cardiac hypertrophy and heart failure

1 Good suggestions might include the following:
- breathlessness or other symptoms that may be attributable to heart failure
- to assess whether previously prescribed loop diuretics are having any beneficial effect
- to assess a heart murmur
- to determine whether treatment of borderline hypertension is justified.

2 True.

3 a True – the relative risk for sudden death is 1.7 for every 50 g/m increment in left ventricular mass.
  b False – it is found in 25% of hypertensives.
  c True.
  d False – echocardiography is better.
  e True – this has been shown in dogs subjected to experimental myocardial ischaemia.
  f True – including angiogram.
  g False – there is no conclusive evidence to date, but there is sufficient suggestive evidence.

4 Six-minute walking test.

5 a True.
  b True – but they need to be introduced gradually.
  c True (whereas other vasodilators generally increase heart rate).
  d False – it has no effect, but other calcium antagonists generally increase heart rate.
  e True.

6 a False – thiazides augment loop diuretics.
  b False – gradual introduction of the ACE inhibitor is a better policy.
  c False – heart failure itself commonly causes cough.
  d True.
  e False – it is of proven benefit.

7 Morphine.

8 a Captopril – 25 mg bd.
  b Enalapril – 10 mg bd.

c Lisinopril – 10 mg od.

d Ramipril – 5 mg bd.

# Arrhythmia

1 a 0.5%.

 b 8.8%.

2 a V1.

 b • Wolff-Parkinson-White syndrome – digoxin or verapamil will accelerate the ventricular response.

  • Sick sinus syndrome – anti-arrhythmic treatment may cause profound brady-cardia, so pacing will be needed before treating the arrhythmia.

3 Holter monitoring is a well-established method, but the patient might need to wear the apparatus for some time before making a recording. Some GPs provide the patient with a letter requesting the casualty department or ECG department to provide an emergency ECG for the bearer immediately on arrival during a bout of palpitations.

 A recent alternative is the Cardiomemo system, in which the patient carries a cassette recorder with a three-point lead which they can place on the chest wall at the onset of palpitations. The recording can be played down a telephone to an ECG technician, who then provides a printout and comments.

4 An echocardiogram might reveal atrial thrombus, indicate the degree of ventricular failure and reveal any structural lesions in the heart.

5 a None at all, except for aspirin or anticoagulants. All anti-arrhythmic treatments have a risk of side-effects which exceeds the benefit in this situation.

 b Digoxin plus a beta-blocker or a calcium antagonist.

 c Digoxin or a low dose of amiodarone.

 d A calcium antagonist.

6 According to the original author the following categories of patient should be referred:

 • those aged < 30 years

 • those with atrial fibrillation that is resistant to the usual drugs for rate control

 • those suitable for cardioversion

 • patients in whom further assessment is needed (e.g. valvular heart disease)

 • those with moderate to severe heart failure

 • those with resistant heart failure

 • those who experience frequent attacks of paroxysmal atrial fibrillation

 • those who experience syncopal attacks due to atrial fibrillation.

7 a All patients with atrial fibrillation which has lasted for more than 48 h.

**b** 2 to 3 weeks.

**c** At least 4 weeks.

**8 a** 14.

   **b** 25.

   **c** 31.

**9 a** True – mitral stenosis increases the risk of embolism by 18-fold.

   **b** False – this is often a short-lived, isolated episode in a healthy heart.

   **c** False – 23% mortality vs. 8% in strokes as a whole, probably because strokes due to atrial fibrillation often involve large total anterior cerebral infarcts.

   **d** True.

**10 a** True.

   **b** False – it is higher.

   **c** False – about 67%.

   **d** True.

   **e** True.

**11** A minority of patients with atrial fibrillation can safely be treated with anticoagulants and will thereafter enjoy a lower risk of embolic stroke. Those with a history of ulcer, bleeding tendency, uncontrolled hypertension, or who cannot comply with blood sampling or treatment are the chief exclusions. However, few practices have a reliable register of all patients with atrial fibrillation. Most of these patients will be taking digoxin or amiodarone, and these can be identified from the repeat-prescribing register on the computer or as they present for repeat prescriptions. Discharge letters from hospital and cardiology clinics provide another possible means of screening for these patients. One doctor suggested that pulse rate and rhythm should be included in the over-75 check, and that if the rhythm appears irregular, the nurse might take a rhythm strip and bring it to the attention of the doctor.

**12 a** Risk of gastrointestinal blood loss – self-report of vomiting blood, or rectal blood loss.

   **b** Risk of haematuria – self-report, check dipstick.

   **c** Alcoholism – more than 28 units per week.

   **d** Using NSAIDs – self-report of regular use, except for prophylactic aspirin.

   **e** Risk of falls – any falls in the past month.

   **f** Inability to use treatment reliably – subject cannot read the label on a bottle of tablets, extract a single tablet, or pick a dose after the strength and colour coding of warfarin tablets have been explained.

   **g** Anaemia – haemoglobin 10 g/dL.

   **h** Coagulation disorder – prothrombin time $> 15$ s.

   **i** Low platelet count – $< 100\,000$.

   **j** Renal failure – serum creatinine $> 300\mu$mol/L.

   **k** Uncontrolled hypertension – $> 180/100$ mmHg.

13 a The recommended range of INR is 2–4, but cautious doctors may prefer not to let the INR rise above 3.5, as the risk of haemorrhage is significantly increased at INRs of > 4.

   b The incidence of stroke was 7.9% per annum in patients on aspirin and a fixed dose of warfarin to produce an INR of 1.3–1.5 to 1.9, but it was only 1.9% in those taking a variable dose of warfarin to produce an INR of > 2.

14 Hypertension, diabetes, or a history of transient ischaemic attacks, stroke or myocardial infarct.

15 a False – approximately 10% of patients produce active metabolites.

   b False – hypothyroidism increases the risk.

   c False – hypokalaemia enhances the risk, but digoxin toxicity may also be related to renal failure, of which hyperkalaemia is a sign.

16 a Cough, fever, dyspnoea and weight loss.

   b Hyperinflation or ground-glass appearance or reticular pattern.

   c Check $FEV_1$ or PFR regularly, monitor the total dose and advise the patient to check for relevant symptoms.

# Miscellaneous

1 a False.

   b True.

   c True.

   d True (almost).

2 a True.

   b False.

   c True.

   d False.

   e True.

   f True.

   g True.

3 Suggestions might include aspirin, vitamin E, folic acid, and avoidance of drugs that prolong QT intervals.

4 Severe malnutrition is associated with a prolonged QT interval, which is a risk factor for ventricular tachyarrhythmias. The association may be mediated by hypokalaemia, and potassium supplements are indicated in such cases.

5 Young men commonly present to their GPs complaining of chest pain. The symptom pattern may suggest a musculoskeletal cause, which will respond to rest and

reassurance that they do not have a cardiac problem. However, the question concerned a combination of breathlessness and chest pain on exercise in a boy whose father had died suddenly while taking strenuous exercise.

Members suggested that a familial tendency to ischaemic heart disease and hypertrophic obstructive cardiomyopathy should be included in the differential diagnosis, as should exercise induced-asthma. The post-mortem report on the father would be useful.

Physical examination after exercise might reveal an outflow tract murmur or a drop in peak flow rate. The response of the symptoms to a GTN tablet or spray would be interesting. ECG evidence of left ventricular hypertrophy or ischaemia could be sought. If suspicion of heart disease remains, or if there is a need for more complete reassurance, referral for echocardiography or possibly an outflow catheter study would be justified.

6   Amiodarone and implanted defibrillator.

7   Mitral valve prolapse. Possible complications include severe mitral reflux, subacute bacterial endocarditis and cerebral thromboembolism.

# Heart attack

1   a The belief that heart attacks usually start with sudden onset of pain, and often with collapse.

b A paramedic should arrive within 8 min at 90% of all calls in all areas.

2   Receptionists need personal tuition in dealing with emergency calls for chest pain. A procedure sheet is insufficient. GPs should ensure that their receptionists know how to get a message to the duty doctor within a minute or two. The receptionist should tell the patient that the message will be transferred to the doctor immediately. If this involves use of a bleep, or if the receptionist knows that the doctor cannot attend to the patient promptly, she should also advise the patient to call an ambulance.

The receptionist should advise the caller to give the patient an aspirin 'to prevent clotting' and a spray or tablet of nitroglycerine if these are available, and to rest in a horizontal position until help is available.

3   Get the patient to casualty as soon as possible because:

• prompt fibrinolysis or precautions against arrhythmia reduce the risk if it is a coronary

• you cannot diagnose a coronary without an ECG, and you have no machine.

Visit because:

• a clear history in familiar circumstances is needed to exclude the possibility of a panic attack

• you can provide pain relief, treatment for arrhythmia, aspirin and a nitrite and (if the diagnosis is a definite myocardial infarction) a thrombolytic before the ambulance will call

- the doctor–patient relationship should be maintained.

The ideal answer is to do both.

4   Urine collected 2–24 h after the onset of chest pain with >1.5 mg albumin/mmol creatinine is likely to come from someone with myocardial infarction. The specificity is 96%, sensitivity is 80% and predictive value is 96%. This concentration of albumin would correspond to approximately 15 mg/L, detectable with microalbuminuria test sticks, but this test would be unreliable in patients with renal disease such as that associated with diabetes.

5   a   False.
    b   False.
    c   True.

6   Aspirin and heparin.

7   False – early administration is not critical. However, the benefit is dependent on treatment being continued for a month or more after the event.

8   Intravenously. If it is given intramuscularly, extensive bruising may occur after administration of thrombolytic drugs.

9   a   False (about 1.6 in 1000).
    b   True.
    c   False.
    d   True (together with aspirin).

10  a   182/344 = 53%.
    b   310/888 = 35%.

11  False – in district general hospitals most patients only receive thrombolytics after admission to the ward or coronary-care unit.

12  In this study, 32% of patients had received an intravenous opiate prior to admission and 68% had received aspirin prior to admission.

13  Aspirin and beta-blockers.

14  Patients who have multiple risk factors, a low exercise capacity, are slow to adjust to a new lifestyle and who have recently had cardiac surgery, and who do not suffer from angina, aortic stenosis or ventricular arrhythmias.

15  32.5%.

# EAR, NOSE AND THROAT

## Otitis media and glue ear

**1** The following factors in a child with otitis media are associated with fever and earache lasting a further 3 days or more: (*True/False*)

**a** onset in winter

**b** age under 2 years

**c** being denied antibiotic treatment.

*BMJ.* **303**:1450–2

**2** What are the sensitivity and specificity of tympanometry when used to assess eardrum mobility in otitis media with effusion, and compared with findings at myringotomy?

*Br J Gen Pract.* **98**: 1079

**3** What is the prognosis for a child with glue ear? (*2 points*)

*BMJ.* **312**: 1517–20 (research report)

**4** Effusion after otitis media: (*True/False*)

**a** is commonest in the second year of life

**b** can be diagnosed with near certainty using microtympanometry.

*BMJ.* **304**: 67–8

**5** Of children with glue ear:

**a** what proportion have been found to have allergic rhinitis?

**b** what proportion have been found to have eosinophilia?

**c** what proportion have been found to have asthma?

**d** what proportion have been found to have eczema?

*BMJ.***306**: 455

**6** What sleeping position may a child adopt to compensate for airway obstruction by enlarged tonsils or adenoids? (*1 point*)

*BMJ.***306**: 640–2

**7** Children with grommets should be allowed to swim. (*True/False*)

*BMJ.***304**: 198

# Nose and sinuses

**1** A patient gives a history of prolonged nasal stuffiness and intermittent facial
pain.
**a** What GP examination technique is best for revealing nasal polyps? (*1 point*)
**b** A trial of what treatment(s) is required before specialist referral is indicated? (*1 point*)
**c** What is the best examination technique available to specialists for revealing deviated nasal septum or nasal polyps?

*BMJ.***308**: 1608–9

**2** Sinusitis. (*True/False*)
**a** The headache may be worse on leaning forward.
**b** The headache is usually worst at night.
**c** Sinusitis may be exacerbated by oral contraceptives.
**d** After inhaling decongestant drops, patients should put their heads back
immediately.

*BMJ.***309**: 1415–21 (review)

**3** The following observations give significant support to a diagnosis of maxillary sinusitis: (*True/False*)
**a** pain on bending forward
**b** anosmia
**c** unilateral pain
**d** unilateral tenderness over the maxillary sinus

**e** raised ESR.

*BMJ.* **311**: 233–5

4 | Nasal polyps. (*True/False*)

**a** They become less prevalent with advancing age.

**b** They usually cause pain.

**c** They commonly cause loss or alteration of the sense of taste.

**d** When drops are applied the nasal cavity should be held below the level of the oropharynx.

**e** A short course of oral steroids can provide rapid relief.

*BMJ.* **311**: 1411–14 (review)

5 | In patients with sinusitis, what median duration of symptoms would you expect if they are assigned to treatment with:

**a** amoxycillin 500 mg tds for 10 days

**b** penicillin 1320 mg tds for 10 days

**c** matching placebo tds for 10 days?

*BMJ.* **313**: 325–8 (trial report)

6 | Doxycycline in the treatment of sinusitis is markedly more effective in relieving symptoms than decongestants and placebo. (*True/False*)

*Br J Gen Pract.* **47**: 794–8 (trial report)

# Vertigo

1 | Patients of average age 60 years who had been dizzy for an average of 2 years were randomized to a control group or to an active group who were taught a programme of exercises to help redevelop their sense of balance.

**a** What proportion of patients in the active and control groups would you expect to feel better after 6 weeks?

**b** Would you expect an independent observer to find evidence of better balance in the treatment group?

*Br J Gen Pract.* **48**: 1136–40 (trial report)

2 | Prescribing a vestibular sedative for a patient with benign positional vertigo is likely to augment the effect of training exercises. (*True/False*)

*BMJ.* **311**: 54 (letter)

**3** Ménière's disease.

  **a** What functional test is useful in cases of doubt about the diagnosis?

  **b** What is the prognosis for balance, and for hearing?

  *BMJ.* **316**: 368–72 (review)

**4** Betahistine (Serc) is contraindicated in peptic ulcer. List three alternative drug therapies for Ménière's disease.

  *BMJ.* **301**: 1532–3

# Miscellaneous

**1** What advice should we give patients on how to minimize the risk of baro-trauma to the ears when flying or when travelling through tunnels? (*4 points*)

  *BMJ.* **309**: 426, 881

**2** How may auriscope earpieces best be sterilized in the GP surgery?

  *BMJ.* **305**: 1571–3

**3** Complications of ear-syringing requiring specialist referral. (*True/False*)

  **a** They occur in about 1 in 300 syringings.

  **b** Failure of wax removal accounts for 30% of referrals.

  **c** Damage to the tympanic membrane or ear canal accounts for about 30% of referrals.

  *BMJ.* **301**: 1251–2

**4** Surfers should wear earplugs. What conditions do they protect against? (*2 points*)

  *BMJ.* **314**: 1918 (citation)

**5** What factors may exacerbate or perpetuate otitis externa? (*5 points*)

  *BMJ.* **315**:1511

**6** Where should an acupuncture needle be inserted in order to relieve nausea? (*1 point*)

  *Br J Gen Pract.* **47**: 47–8 (discussion paper)

**7** Acoustic neuroma. (*True/False*)

a Deafness to low-pitched sounds is characteristic.

b Distortion rather than loss of hearing is characteristic.

c A feeling of pressure in the ear is characteristic.

d Ataxia is often the first neurological symptom.

e Pure-tone audiometry is a useful screening tool in a patient with suspect symptoms.

*BMJ.* **311**: 1141–4 (review)

# Deafness

**1** Screening the elderly for hearing impairment. (*True/False*)

a In patients aged 65 years or over the prevalence of hearing loss that would justify provision of a hearing-aid is around 10%.

b About 75% of elderly patients who are found to justify the use of an NHS hearing-aid want to have one.

*Br J Gen Pract.* **43**: 406–8

**2** Which deaf patients may benefit from cochlear implantation? (*2 points*)

*BMJ.* **311**: 1588 (editorial)

**3** What are the advantages of digital hearing aids? (*2 points*)

*BMJ.* **315**: 354–7 (review)

# Tinnitus

**1** 'I've got ringing in my ears, doctor.' List four or more questions that the doctor may ask to elicit causal factors. (*4 points*)

*BMJ.* **306**: 1490–1

*BMJ.* **307**: 262

**2** Which patients with tinnitus require specialist referral, and which specialties are most appropriate for them?

*BMJ.* **302**: 1267

**3** What forms of therapy may make tinnitus more bearable? (*6 or more points*)

*BMJ.* **308**: 1238

*BMJ.* **314**: 729–31 (review)

# Sore throats

**1** The following findings in a patient with a sore throat suggest infection with streptococci:

**a** swollen posterior lymph nodes

**b** cough

**c** fever

**d** duration of more than 3 days

**e** exudate on the tonsils.

*Br J Gen Pract.* **41**: 504–7

# ANSWERS

## Otitis media and glue ear

1   a  False – the illness is just as prolonged if it is contracted in summer.

    b  True – younger children often develop the condition particularly severely.

    c  False – there is little evidence that antibiotics speed the cure significantly.

2   Sensitivity is 90% and specificity is 86%.

3   50% of cases will resolve within 3 months and 75% within 6 months.

4   a  False – it is commonest at 6–12 months.

    b  False – 30% of those cases diagnosed were found to have no fluid at operation.

5   a  80%.

    b  35%.

    c  >35%.

    d  20%. These figures support the conclusion that glue ear is more a problem of allergy than one of infection.

6   Resting on the knees and elbows with the neck hyperextended.

7   True.

## Nose and sinuses

1   a  Anterior rhinoscopy with the auroscope.

    b  Intranasal steroids. Possibly also use antihistamines or antibiotics in suitable cases.

    c  Nasal endoscopy.

2   a  True.

    b  False.

    c  True.

    d  False.

3   a  False – this had no predictive value for mucopurulent antral aspirate in patients with suspected maxillary sinusitis.

    b  False – any predictive effect of this sign did not reach the level of statistical significance.

    c  True – this only just reached the level of statistical significance.

d True – this definitely has predictive value.

e True – ESR over 10 mm/h in men or over 20 mm/h in women and C-reactive protein over 10 mg/L in either sex were both predictive of purulent antral aspirate in these patients.

4    a False – their prevalence increases with age.

b False – they are usually painless.

c True – loss of sense of smell is constant, and is usually accompanied by loss or alteration of taste.

d True.

e True.

5    a 8 days.

b 10 days.

c 15 days – from the results of a clinical trial.

6    False – from the results of the trial reported in the reference.

# Vertigo

1    a 54% in the treatment group and 28% in the control group rated themselves as feeling better after 6 weeks.

b The observer found significantly better performance on testing ability to maintain a heel-to-toe position in the treatment group after 6 months.

2    False – it may prevent the habituation from the training exercises.

3    a After glycerol dehydration, patients with Ménière's disease and the occasional patient with endolymphatic hydrops can be shown to have improved acuity for low tones on audiometry.

b Paroxysms of rocking or rotatory vertigo get worse, but after a period they diminish, although the patient commonly remains unsteady, particularly in the dark. Sensorineural hearing loss, initially affecting only the lower tones, fluctuates initially but later it steadily worsens, and both ears are usually affected.

4    • Diuretic and salt restriction.

• Vestibular sedatives such as cinnarizine or prochlorperazine.

• Vasodilators such as nicotinic acid.

# Miscellaneous

1    Increases in ambient pressure on descent from the sky or into tunnels, or when a passing train approaches in a tunnel, can cause acute pain and occasional rupture of the tympanic membrane when the eustachian tube is blocked. Patients with catarrh or rhinitis are particularly prone to the problem, and those who have undergone stapedectomy in the previous 2 months are best advised not to use these means of transport.

    Countermeasures suggested by members included using steam inhalations before travel, the use of menthol and other decongestants during travel, and repeated exercises to maintain the patency of the eustachian tube immediately before and during take-off and descent. On a flight, descent may be heralded by a reduction in engine noise before the captain advises the passengers. The Valsalva manoeuvre, sucking sweets and the Frenzel manoeuvre (repetitive movements of the tongue against the soft palate) were all described as suitable exercises in the original article. One member also mentioned that flights into airports that demand a steep angle of descent (e.g. London Docklands) are particularly likely to cause trouble. Air hostesses sometimes block their ear canals with Blu-Tack or cotton wool soaked in Vaseline on descent, or apply a hot cup or a hot flannel with an airtight seal around the ear on descent, in order to maintain higher pressure in the ear canal.

2    Recommended methods are autoclaving, boiling for 5 min or soaking in 70% alcohol or other disinfectant for 5 min.

3    a  False – they occur in about 1 in 1000 syringings.

      b  True – in resistant cases Exterol, which contains hydrogen peroxide, appears to be the most effective wax softener.

      c  True – the syringe should not be pointed directly at the tympanic membrane. An alternative method of removing the wax is indicated if there is otitis media or externa or a previously perforated eardrum, or if the ear containing the wax is the only hearing ear.

4    Otitis externa and surfer's ear, i.e. new bone laid down in the ear canal, leading to stenosis.

5    Underlying eczema or psoriasis, immunodeficiency (e.g. diabetes), drug-resistant organisms, sensitivity to treatment (e.g. neomycin), perichondritis, and scratching leading to dermatitis artefacta.

6    At point P6 – two thumb-breadths proximal to the palmar crease on the right forearm, in the midline of the palmar surface. The same point is pressed upon by a stud in a wrist cuff in commercially available remedies for seasickness.

7    a  False – high-tone deafness is characteristic.

      b  True.

c True.

d True.

e True.

# Deafness

1 a False – the prevalence of hearing loss that would justify a hearing-aid is of the order of 30%.

  b False – uptake in the elderly is approximately 50%.

2 • Adults with total bilateral loss of hearing after acquiring speech and language.

  • Children born deaf or who become deaf before learning spoken language, and who receive the implant before reaching the age of 7 years.

    The danger in other groups is that partial reliance on hearing through a cochlear implant will impair the development of skill in using communication systems for the deaf.

3 The signal can be processed to suppress noise or to amplify specific frequencies, and the most recently developed ones can tune themselves automatically to human speech. They are also easier to handle.

# Tinnitus

1 • One ear or both? Unilateral tinnitus may be a marker for acoustic neuroma.

  • Is your hearing dull? This common associated feature suggests cochlear disorder.

  • Does anyone else observe the ringing when you are close to them?

  • How is life treating you? Are you feeling OK otherwise? Stress may aggravate perception of tinnitus.

  • What medicines are you taking? Aspirin or quinine may be contributory factors if taken at high dose, or if drug metabolism or excretion is impaired.

2 • Patients who find the tinnitus intolerable may benefit from referral to an audiologist for consideration for a masking device and for a detailed discussion of the problem.

  • Those with features suggestive of cerebral tumour may benefit from early referral to a neurologist.

  • Those with prominent secondary psychological symptoms may benefit from referral to a psychiatrist or clinical psychologist or community psychiatric nurse.

3 Cognitive therapy, hypnotherapy, relaxation therapy, biofeedback, manipulation of diet, ultrasound, masking devices, hearing aids, antidepressants, tranquillizers and sedatives. Some authorities also maintain that betahistine is worthy of trial.

# Sore throats

1 a False.
  b False.
  c True.
  d False.
  e True.

# GASTROENTEROLOGY

## Dyspepsia, ulcers and *Helicobacter pylori*

**1** Atrophic gastritis.

  **a** What infection appears to be commonly associated with atrophic gastritis in the elderly?

  **b** What drug treatment may combine with this infection to cause atrophic gastritis in one third of those who had the combination?

  *BMJ.* **312**: 648 (citation)

  *BMJ.* **313**: 250 (news item)

**2** *Helicobacter pylori.* (*True/False*)

  **a** Infection is associated with social deprivation.

  **b** Serological diagnosis can be made from saliva.

  *BMJ.* **309**: 1119–23

**3** The following subjects are much more likely than not to have a gastric infection with *Helicobacter pylori*: (*True/False*)

  **a** a patient aged less than 60 years with recurring or chronic dyspepsia

  **b** a patient with chronic dyspepsia with gastritis observed on gastroscopy

  **c** a patient with chronic dyspepsia with peptic ulcer observed on gastroscopy.

  *BMJ.* **304**: 1276–94

**4** Dyspepsia. (*True/False*)

  **a** Patients with a past history of epigastric pain are more likely to have endoscopic evidence of peptic ulcer disease than of oesophagitis.

**b** Patients with a past complaint of heartburn are more likely to have peptic ulcer disease demonstrated on endoscopy than are controls.

*BMJ.* **302**: 749–52

**5** What prevalence of *Helicobacter pylori* infection identified by breath tests would you expect in patients aged 15–79 years attending a general practice in the following categories?

**a** Do not drink coffee.

**b** Drink three or more cups of coffee per day.

**c** Do not drink alcohol.

**d** Drink 75 g or more of alcohol per day.

*BMJ.* **315**:1489–92 (research report)

**6** Which of the following patients should have an upper GI endoscopy? In each case state a reason for your point of view.

**a** A woman aged 38 years with intermittent epigastric pain relieved by eating, for 2 weeks after taking non-steroidal drugs for back pain for the previous month.

**b** Food sticks in the lower oesophagus in a 35-year-old man every 10 days or so when he bolts his meals without chewing.

**c** A 30-year-old man with epigastric pain every night for the past 2 weeks, that is relieved by antacids, who smokes 20 cigarettes per day and drinks heavily.

*BMJ.* **310**: 853–6

**7** The following advice on management of dyspepsia and *H.pylori* infection is backed by firm evidence. (*True/False*)

**a** Patients with long-term dyspepsia should be screened for *H. pylori* antibodies.

**b** All patients newly diagnosed with gastric or duodenal ulceration should receive eradication therapy.

**c** Patients with persisting dyspepsia after eradication therapy should have a urease breath test.

**d** Patients who have not responded to previous eradication therapy should be treated with bismuth 120 mg qds, metronidazole 400 mg tds and tetracycline 500 mg qds or with omeprazole 20 mg bd, amoxycillin 500 mg qds and metronidazole for 14 days.

*Br J Gen Pract.* **45**: 489–92 (review)

**8** The following are representative estimates of costings, prevalences, test validities and cure rates relevant to peptic ulcer disease. Can you use them to devise a reasonable policy and estimate the cost-effectiveness of two policies of your own choosing for management of dyspepsia in temperate, non-smoking patients aged under 45 years who do not use NSAIDs?

*Estimates*
In temperate, non-smoking patients who do not use NSAIDs, aged under 45 years, newly presenting with 4 weeks of antacid-responsive dyspepsia

| | |
|---|---|
| • prevalence of carriage of *H. pylori* | 40% |
| • prevalence of peptic ulcer if *H. pylori* is present | 25% |
| • prevalence of peptic ulcer if *H. pylori* is absent | 3% |
| • prevalence of gastro-oesophageal reflux | 20% |
| • prevalence of gastric carcinoma | negligible |

*Costs*

| | |
|---|---|
| • a GP consultation | £8 |
| • a consultant consultation | £39 |
| • *Helicobacter* antibody test | £13 |
| • urease breath test | £31 |
| • endoscopy and CLO test | £76 |
| • 1 month of treatment with simple antacid | £5 |
| • 1 month of treatment with compound antacid | £10 |
| • 1 month of treatment with high-dose $H_2$ antagonist | £21 |
| • 1 month of treatment with low-dose $H_2$ antagonist | £10 |
| • 1 month of treatment with proton-pump inhibitor | £35 |
| • eradication therapy for *H. pylori* | £38 |

*Predictive validity of tests*

| | |
|---|---|
| • serology for *H. pylori* | 70% |
| • endoscopy and CLO test for *H. pylori* | 100% |
| • urease breath test for *H. pylori* | 85% |

*Cure or control rates*

| | |
|---|---|
| • eradication therapy for *H. pylori* | 85% |
| • effective control of simple dyspepsia with: | |
|    – simple antacid | 70% |
|    – compound antacid | 75% |
|    – $H_2$ antagonist, low dose | 95% |
|    – proton-pump inhibitor | 100% |

- effective control of peptic ulcer with:
  - simple antacid                                                30%
  - compound antacid                                          35%
  - $H_2$ antagonist, high dose for 1 month, then low dose    75%
  - proton-pump inhibitor                                        95%
- effective control of gastro-oesophageal reflux with:
  - simple antacid                                                20%
  - compound antacid                                          33%
  - $H_2$ antagonist                                             50%
  - proton-pump inhibitor                                        90%

*Reinfection rate with* H. pylori                                1% per year

*Recurrence rate of peptic ulcer in the first year:*
- *H. pylori* present, maintenance $H_2$ antagonist             40%
- *H. pylori* present, no maintenance $H_2$ antagonist          70%
- *H. pylori* absent, maintenance H antagonist                 1%
- *H. pylori* absent, no maintenance H antagonist              5%

*Number of GP consultations required per year if patient has:*
- persistent non-ulcer dyspepsia                               4
- inadequately treated peptic ulcer                            6
- inadequately treated gastro-oesophageal reflux              5

*Days of discomfort per year if patient has:*
- persistent non-ulcer dyspepsia                               40
- inadequately treated peptic ulcer                            160
- inadequately treated gastro-oesophageal reflux              100

*Average economic value of a day of discomfort*                £20

BMJ. **312**: 1321–5 (economic research report), 1361– 2 (letters)

**9** Dyspepsia.

**a** How many of 165 dyspeptic patients with no ulcer at initial endoscopy developed one over 10 years of follow-up?

**b** Prokinetic drugs are as effective as $H_2$-blockers in treating the symptoms of ulcer-like dyspepsia in the absence of peptic ulcer on endoscopy. (*True/False*)

**c** What prevalence of peptic ulcer has been found in patients with the following as predominant symptoms:

　i  heartburn, dyspepsia and acid regurgitation

ii localized epigastric pain, pain when hungry and pain relieved by food or antacids that wakens the patient from sleep, and remits and relapses

iii upper abdominal discomfort often aggravated by food, with early satiety, postprandial fullness, nausea, retching or vomiting, and bloating?

**d** i What are the benefits of endoscopy for a patient with dyspepsia in whom there is no significant risk of stomach cancer?

ii Do these benefits justify endoscopy in the absence of *Helicobacter* antibodies?

iii Do these benefits justify endoscopy in the presence of *Helicobacter* antibodies and a response to a triple therapy for *Helicobacter*?

iv Do these benefits justify endoscopy in the presence of *Helicobacter* antibodies but no symptomatic response to triple therapy?

**e** In an age group where the prevalence of *Helicobacter pylori* in the stomach is 25%, what is the percentage probability that a patient is harbouring *Helicobacter* if:

i a rapid whole blood test for *Helicobacter* antibodies with a good sensitivity to specificity ratio is positive

ii a laboratory ELISA kit with average sensitivity is positive

iii a urea breath test is positive?

*BMJ.* **315**: 1284–7 (review)

**10** After eradication therapy for *H. pylori*, patients with persisting dyspeptic symptoms are likely to have a persistent positive $^{13}$C-urea breath test. (*True/False*)

*BMJ.* **312**: 349 (research report)

**11** A patient with dyspepsia and who is positive for *H. pylori* on a urea breath test reports no diminution of symptoms after a course of triple therapy for *H. pylori*. What are the further diagnostic possibilities and how will you now manage the problem?

*BMJ.* **316**: 162–3 (leading article)

**12** An elderly patient has previously been shown on gastroscopy to have gastritis or a benign ulcer, and to respond to medical treatment. If the dyspepsia recurs, after what interval from the previous endoscopy should he undergo further endoscopy to rule out gastric or oesophageal cancer? (*2 or more points*)

*BMJ.* **314**: 467–71 (research report and discussion)

**13** Treatment to eradicate *H. pylori* is recommended as soon as a peptic ulcer is discovered in a patient with severe dyspepsia. (*True/False*)

*BMJ.* **302**: 919–20

**14** What reduction in the use of acid suppressant treatment can be expected from providing triple therapy for patients with dyspepsia who are positive on testing for *H. pylori* antibodies?

*Br J Gen Pract.* **47**: 660 (letter)

**15** a What serum assay should be undertaken in a patient with recurrent peptic ulcers, despite being a non-smoker with no *Helicobacter coli* in a mucosal sample at a recent endoscopy? (*1 point*)

b What conditions should be observed at the time of sampling? (*3 points*)

*BMJ.* **306**: 1728–31

**16** In reflux oesophagitis, what percentage success rates are typical for the following treatments?

a Ranitidine.

b Ranitidine plus cisapride.

c Omeprazole.

*BMJ.* **307**: 456

**17** What cumulative incidence of gastrointestinal haemorrhage was found in this study to be associated with taking aspirin to prevent thrombosis?

*BMJ.* **311**: 1312 (citation)

**18** A patient with dyspepsia would benefit from anticoagulant treatment. What can be done to reduce the risks? (*2 or more points*)

*BMJ.* **310**: 1118

**19** The presence of stomach acid reduces the risk of salmonella gastroenteritis. (*True/False*)

*BMJ.* **308**: 176

**20** What are the likely effects of chronic vomiting on the serum levels of the following electrolytes?

a Chloride.

b Sodium.

**c** Bicarbonate.

*BMJ.* **309**: 592

---

**21** In a patient seen at home with haematemesis, and known to have a history of peptic ulcer: (*True/False*)

**a** an immediate injection of an $H_2$ antagonist is likely to improve the prognosis

**b** an immediate injection of tranexamic acid is likely to improve the prognosis

**c** long-term treatment with beta-blockers is likely to reduce the risk of recurrence.

*BMJ.* **304**: 135–6

---

**22** Non-steroidal anti-inflammatory drugs and peptic ulcer. (*True/False*)

**a** The use of NSAIDs for a few weeks only in the elderly is quite safe.

**b** Giving NSAIDs in parenteral or rectal form has been shown to reduce the risk.

*BMJ.* **310**: 817–18

---

**23** The following drugs may be useful for relieving hypomotility of the stomach: (*True/False*)

**a** hyoscine

**b** erythromycin

**c** goserelin

**d** a tricyclic antidepressant

**e** bethanechol.

*BMJ.* **310**: 308–11

---

**24** By what percentage does misoprostol reduce the risk of serious gastrointestinal complications in patients taking NSAIDs? (*1 point*)

*BMJ.* **311**:1518–19 (editorial)

---

**25** Somatostatin is reported to help in the following disorders: (*True/False*)

**a** bleeding from oesophageal varices

**b** bleeding peptic ulcer

**c** acute pancreatitis

**d** dumping syndrome

**e** secretory diarrhoea.

*BMJ.* **44**: 1381–2

# Bowel disorders

**1** How should rebound tenderness be elicited?

*BMJ.* **305**: 44–6

**2** Constipation.

**a** How would you differentiate a colonic tumour from a constipated colon on physical examination? (*3 points*)

**b** By what mechanisms may cancer cause constipation? (*5 points*)

**c** What seems to be the best treatment for the following problems:

   i  soft stools in a lax rectum (*1 point*)

   ii  hard stools limited to the rectum (*2 points*)

   iii  faecal impaction extending deep into the colon. (*2 points*)

**d** What particular requirement is needed when treating constipation in a patient with a stoma? (*1 point*)

**e** What unusual appearance may be noted by patients who take danthron? (*1 point*)

*BMJ.* **315**: 1293–6 (review)

**3** What blood tests are useful for identifying cases of toxocariasis? (*3 points*)

*BMJ.* **309**: 5–6

**4** Defining the irritable bowel syndrome. (*True/False*)

**a** Abdominal pain must always be present.

**b** Abdominal pain must be relieved by defaecation.

**c** Mucus in the stools is an essential feature.

**d** Straining at stool may be a feature.

**e** A sense of incomplete evacuation may be a feature.

*BMJ.* **314**: 779–82 (research report)

**5** Irritable bowel syndrome. (*True/False*)

**a** A small minority of patients with IBS respond to an exclusion diet consisting of one meat, one carbohydrate and one fruit.

**b** Post-dysenteric IBS rarely responds to drug treatment.

**c** Diagnosis in a young adult should be by exclusion after multiple investigations.

**d** A selective serotonin reuptake inhibitor (SSRI) would be the appropriate type of antidepressant for a depressed IBS sufferer with diarrhoea.

*BMJ.* **309**: 1646–8 (discussion papers)

**6** The following conditions are associated with irritable bowel syndrome. (*True/ False*)

**a** Migraine.

**b** Wheeze.

**c** Bladder detrusor instability.

**d** Rectal bleeding.

*BMJ.* **304**: 87–90

**7** Which antibody test has 100% predictive value for villous atrophy and clinical improvement on withdrawing gluten?

*BMJ.* **303**: 1163–5

**8** Evidence suggests that patients with coeliac disease or dermatitis herpetiformis can take up to 50 g of oats per day for 12 weeks without suffering relapse. (*True/False*)

*BMJ.* **313**: 1300–1 (research report)

*BMJ.* **314**: 159–60 (leading article)

**9** What 10-year recurrence rate for Crohn's disease has been found:

**a** in smokers

**b** in non-smokers?

*BMJ.* **313**: 265–6 (survey report)

**10** What dietary management can be of benefit to patients with Crohn's disease? (*2 points*)

*BMJ.* **310**: 113-15 (review)

**11** Malabsorption of what nutrient is found in up to 60% of people with Crohn's disease?

*BMJ.* **314**: 1552 (correspondence)

**12** Fish oil improves the prognosis for Crohn's disease in remission. (*True/False*)

*BMJ.* **312**: 1682 (citation)

**13** Management of ulcerative colitis. (*True/False*)

  **a** What is an appropriate dose of prednisolone for a relapse?

  **b** What percentage of patients do not tolerate salazopyrin?

  **c** If 5-aminosalicylates fail to prevent frequent relapses, what other treatment may be used for this purpose?

  *BMJ.* **305**: 35–7

**14** Colitis due to *Clostridium difficile* : (*True/False*)

  **a** commonly causes symptoms in infants

  **b** usually presents as a bloody diarrhoea

  **c** can be treated with broad-spectrum penicillins.

  *BMJ.* **310**: 1375–80

**15** A 45-year-old man tells you that his father died of carcinoma of the colon. What will you suggest to reduce his risk of a similar fate? (*2 points*)

  *BMJ.* **306**: 707

  *BMJ.* **307**: 277–9

**16** Why may a sedentary job protect against rectal cancer? (*1 point*)

  *BMJ.* **307**: 1368

**17** Screening for asymptomatic colorectal cancer.

  **a** What family history of the disorder would justify sending a young or middle-aged person for screening? (*3 points*)

  **b** What screening tests appear to be worth performing in subjects with hereditary non-polyposis colorectal cancer syndrome? (*7 points*)

  **c** What proportion of the general population will develop colonic cancer?

  **d** Results of screening using faecal occult blood. (*quote ranges*)

   i What proportion of subjects proceed to colonoscopy?

   ii What difference is there between control and screened subjects in the proportion of cancers detected at stage A?

   iii What decrease in cancer-related mortality has been reported?

   iv What compliance rates are reported?

  **e** What dietary restrictions are required to prevent false-positive results when testing for faecal occult blood?

  **f** What reduction in death rates from distal colorectal carcinoma is suggested from case–control studies of screening the normal population using flexible sigmoidoscopy?

*BMJ.* **314**: 285–90

**18** When screening patients aged 45–64 years with Haemoccult for faecal occult blood: (*True/False*)

**a** a 3% yield of positive results in compliers can be expected

**b** of patients with a positive result ,the majority are also positive when the test is repeated while they are on a restricted diet

**c** most patients who receive unsolicited test kits from their doctor use them and return them.

*Br J Gen Pract.* **42**: 18–20

**19** On inviting 3509 patients aged 50–80 years to take part in screening with Haemoccult:

**a** how many patients with a colonic adenoma are likely to be identified

**b** how many patients with a colorectal carcinoma are likely to be identified?

*Br J Gen Pract.* **46**: 283–6 (research report)

**20** By how much has testing people aged 45–64 years for faecal occult blood every 2 years reduced the death rate from colon cancer?

*BMJ.* **313**: 1425 (news item)

**21** Gastrointestinal investigation of iron deficiency anaemia. (*True/False*)

**a** Pathology on examining the upper gastrointestinal tract is found in more than 20% of cases of colonic cancer.

**b** In the absence of colonic symptoms, a finding of oesophagitis or gastric erosion in an elderly patient is sufficient explanation for the anaemia.

**c** Colonoscopy is more likely than double-contrast barium enema to identify a tumour of the ascending colon.

*BMJ.* **314**: 206–8 (research report)

**22** A tumour of the ascending colon is most likely to present with pain, altered bowel habit or acute obstruction. (*True/False*)

*BMJ.* **304**: 1651–3

**23** Can you devise a policy on which patients presenting with rectal bleeding require sigmoidoscopy or colonoscopy? (*2 or more points*)

*Br J Gen Pract.* **46**: 161–3

*BMJ.* **304**: 1521–2

**24** According to a recent consensus statement, how frequently should a patient with multiple colonic polyps undergo follow-up colonoscopy?

*BMJ.* **303**: 3–4

**25** What blood test seems likely to be of value in screening patients who have had a colorectal cancer removed for recurrence? (*1 point*)

*Br J Gen Pract.* **45**: 3, 287–8

**26** A patient is shortly to go for a colonoscopy. What advice will you give on precautions while using the preliminary purgative?

*BMJ.* **314**: 74 (letters)

**27** For what bowel condition may inhalation of salbutamol be a suitable treatment?

*BMJ.* **312**: 1682 (citation)

**28** How might you advise a sufferer from proctalgia fugax to relieve the condition without use of medication?

*BMJ.* **305**: 243–6

**29** In the management of anal disorders: (*True/False*)
**a** a proctoscope is needed to visualize an anal fissure
**b** antibiotics are the only treatment required for most perianal abscesses.

*BMJ.* **304**: 904–6

**30** Why does twice daily application of 0.2–0.8% glyceryl trinitrate ointment for 6 weeks lead to healing of most anal fissures and ulcers? (*1 point*)

*BMJ.* **314**: 1638–9 (leading article)

# ANSWERS

## Dyspepsia, ulcers and *Helicobacter pylori*

1  a  *Helicobacter pylori.*
   b  Proton-pump inhibitors.

2  a  True.
   b  True.

3  a  False.
   b  False.
   c  True.

4  a  False – the nature of dyspeptic symptoms is a poor predictor of findings on gastroscopy.
   b  True.

5  a and b  Drinking three or more cups of coffee per day was associated with a prevalence of 28%, whereas non-coffee-drinkers had a prevalence of 12%.
   c and d  Drinking 75 g of alcohol or more per week was associated with a prevalence of 15%, whereas teetotallers had a prevalence of 23%.

6  a  In the case of the 38-year-old woman with intermittent epigastric pain, relieved by eating, for 2 weeks after taking non-steroidal drugs for back pain for the previous month, several members thought that this patient would be best advised to change to a conventional analgesic. The question of whether an endoscopy is indicated could be reviewed after 2 weeks. She might also be advised to use antacids and to take an $H_2$ antagonist if she ever required anti-inflammatory drugs in the future. An endoscopy would have the advantage of identifying any ulcer and *Helicobacter pylori* carried by this patient that might justify a course of acid-suppressing and antibiotic treatment. However, this could be delayed until the effects of adjusting her treatment had been assessed.

   b  In the case of the 35-year-old man in whom food sticks in the throat every 10 days or so when he bolts his meals without chewing, most doctors answering this question thought that this problem was most probably due to a motility disorder in the patient's oesophagus, which would be more likely to show up on a barium swallow than on an endoscopy. If the problem is intermittent and not progressive, investigation would probably be unnecessary and the patient might appreciate advice on taking fluids with every meal, and eating more slowly.

   c  In the case of the 30-year-old man who experienced epigastric pain every night for 2 weeks relieved by antacids, who smokes 20 cigarettes per day and drinks heavily, most doctors answering this question thought that this patient's symptoms should be used to encourage him to modify his lifestyle. If the problem persisted, an endoscopy might be needed to identify whether he has an ulcer or an infection with *H. pylori*.

7  a  False.

   b  True.

   c  True.

   d  True.

8  Doctors answering this question based their answers on managing 100 non-smoking patients aged under 45 years who are moderate drinkers and have suffered dyspepsia for several weeks.

Investigating cases of dyspepsia with a urea breath test and providing eradication therapy for those who showed evidence of *Helicobactor pylori* infection, while providing $H_2$ antagonists for those who did not, would result in a first-year bill of £13 489. If instead those who tested negative were treated with a simple antacid for dyspepsia or a compound antacid for reflux, the cost would be £10 965 in the first year.

To arrange an *H. pylori* antibody test, provide eradication treatment if positive, or use the $H_2$ antagonist if negative,  would cost £14 391 in the first year.

To treat with a high-dose $H_2$ antagonist for 1 month, then switch to a lower dose, arrange endoscopy if symptoms persist and, if treatment fails, to arrange endoscopy would costed £12 800 in the first year.

To undertake endoscopy and biopsy at presentation, provide eradication therapy if *H. pylori* positive and, if there was no resolution to continue with a proton-pump inhibitor, would cost £8520 in the first year. To provide cimetidine for 1 month, then undertake endoscopy and biopsy, provide eradication therapy if *H. pylori* positive and, if there was no resolution, to continue with a proton-pump inhibitor, would cost £3437 in the first year.

A comparison of immediate endoscopy and CLO test compared to initial screening with serology followed by endoscopy if positive favoured the first policy.

Correspondence relating to the original article can be found in the *British Medical Journal* (**313**: 622–3). Interesting conclusions reached by these correspondents are listed below.

• Eradication therapy based on serology alone compares unfavourably with initially using symptomatic treatment, starting with antacids, and progressing to more expensive $H_2$ antagonists and then PPIs if necessary. The cost of endoscopy is around £127 to £300, not £76 as previously quoted.

• American studies have shown that there is little to choose between early endoscopy and initial empirical treatment with antacids or antisecretory drugs.

• Leaving HP untreated may result in later gastric cancer and coronary heart disease, but treating it inadequately is already being associated with the emergence of resistant strains.

In everyday practice the appropriate management policy will depend on the length of waiting time for gastroscopy, the age of the patient (which is related to the prevalence of *H. pylori*) and the patient's own preference.

An expert group at one health agency has concluded that for patients under 40 years of age with dyspepsia unexplained by lifestyle, the best approach is to give cimetidine at the first attendance, arrange an antibody study, and provide eradication therapy if it is positive. Only if symptoms persist should GPs request endoscopy. This approach is supported by little direct validation as yet, but it does seem likely to provide maximal benefit with minimal invasiveness and cost.

9  a  Four of 165 with dyspepsia but no ulcer at the initial endoscopy had ulcer identified over the next 10 years.

   b  True.

   c  i  11%.

      ii  9%.

      iii  7%.

   d  i  An endoscopy will demonstrate whether an ulcer, gastro-oesophageal reflux disease (GORD) and/or *H. pylori* are present. It is valuable to reassure the patient. Clinical trials have shown that patients who undergo endoscopy have lower drug consumption thereafter, lose less time from work and visit their GP less often.

      ii  Endoscopy is justified to demonstrate ulcer, GORD and *H. pylori*. The sensitivity of the enzyme-linked immunosorbent assay has been quoted as around 85% and that of the whole blood test is about 90%.

      iii  Empirical treatment is probably better in this group unless endoscopy is readily available.

      iv  Endoscopy is necessary for reassurance and to identify ulcer, GORD and *H. pylori*.

   e  i  69%.

      ii  57%.

      iii  89%.

10  True – in patients who were breath-test negative 1 and 6 months after treatment the prevalence of symptoms (epigastric discomfort, heartburn, nausea, vomiting or wind) was 12.5% at 1 month and 2.5% at 6 months. If the breath test was positive the prevalence was 56% at 1 month and 91% at 6 months. Thus persisting dyspepsia after treatment for *Helicobacter* based on a firm diagnosis is likely to be due to inadequate eradication.

11  The most likely cause of persisting dyspepsia is inadequate eradication of *H. pylori*. However, one should also consider gastro-oesophageal reflux if this has not already been ruled out, and also gallstones, so the patient may benefit from an ultrasound examination.

12  Dyspepsia in people over 40 years of age necessitates gastroscopy to rule out stomach cancer. However, if no cancer is found one wonders for how long this finding remains valid should symptoms return. Doubling times for gastric cancer have been estimated at anything from 2 months to 10 years, so there is little guidance there. Most members estimated that 6 to 12 months would be a suitable interval between follow-up

gastroscopies, the lower figure being more relevant to patients aged over 60 years and those whose symptoms include early satiety, dysphagia or weight loss, and perhaps longer intervals being appropriate in those who have already undergone two or more gastroscopies. A study of the diagnostic yield from repeat gastroscopies would make interesting reading.

13 False – preliminary treatment with an acid-suppressing regime until dyspepsia is controlled is likely to reduce the risk of intolerable side-effects from the antibiotics.

14 Use of acid-suppressing treatment was approximately halved in this study in one general practice. Only seven of 13 such patients collected prescriptions for acid-suppressing treatment in the 3 months after taking triple therapy to eradicate *H. pylori*.

15 a Serum gastrin. The patient should be fasting, should not have used a protein-pump inhibitor for the previous 2 weeks and should not have used an $H_2$ antagonist for the previous 3 days. The sample should be taken at the laboratory, as gastrin is very unstable, and the sample should be treated immediately to prevent it from decomposing.

   b The urea electrolytes and calcium levels should also be checked.

16 a 50%.

   b 83%.

   c 90%.

17 Approximately 2%.

18 Test for and eliminate *Helicobacter pylori* if it is found. Perform endoscopy for a precise diagnosis and use antisecretory drugs if indicated.

19 True.

20 a Chloride reduced.

   b Sodium reduced.

   c Bicarbonate increased.

21 a False.

   b True.

   c False – but it would if the bleeding was due to oesophageal varices.

22 a False – bleeds are particularly likely in the early weeks of treatment.

   b False.

23 a False.

   b True.

   c True.

   d False.

   e True.

24 40%.

25 a True.

b False.

c False.

d True.

e True.

# Bowel disorders

1 By percussion of a warm finger laid on several places on the abdomen – starting at a point at some distance from the painful area and working towards it.

2 a Indentability, lack of local tenderness and mobility of the mass suggest constipation, whereas the opposite observations suggest a tumour. Malodorous breath and faecal leakage also suggest constipation.

b Use of opiates, gastrointestinal obstruction, immobility, local pain, cord compression, or a cauda equina lesion which abolishes the anocolonic reflex.

c   i An oral stimulant laxative.

ii A glycerine suppository, followed up with oral treatment.

iii A lubricant enema such as arachis oil delivered high into the sigmoid colon, perhaps using a Foley catheter with the balloon dilated for 10 min to prevent leakage back, followed next morning by a phosphate enema. The procedure may need to be repeated several times and followed by oral treatment to prevent recurrence.

d No sphincter exists, so the suppositories need to be held in place with a gloved finger, and enemas may need to be retained by dilating a Foley catheter for 10 min.

e The urine turns pink.

3 • Differential WBC for eosinophilia.

• Immunoglobulin levels – for raised IgE.

• *Toxocara* antibodies.

• Isohaemagglutinins.

4 a True.

b False – alternatively pain may be associated with a change in frequency or consistency of stool.

c False – it is one of five features, of which three must be present for 2 or more days per week.

d True.

e True.

The irritable bowel syndrome is defined as follows.

Abdominal pain relieved by defaecation or associated with a change in frequency or consistency of stool and irregular pattern of defaecation for at least 2 days a week with three or more of the following:

- altered stool frequency
- altered stool form (hard/loose)
- altered stool passage (straining/urgency/sense of incomplete evacuation)
- mucus per rectum
- bloating or feeling of abdominal distension.

5 a False – slightly less than half of IBS sufferers respond to an exclusion diet.

b False (may respond to cholestyramine, aluminium hydroxide or loperamide).

c False.

d False – a tricyclic antidepressant might reduce diarrhoea, whereas an SSRI may worsen bowel symptoms.

6 a True.

b False.

c True.

d True.

7 The IgA antibody to gliadin was found to have 100% predictive value in this study.

8 True.

9 a 70%.

b 41%.

10 An elemental diet and an exclusion diet have both been found to be helpful in controlled trials.

11 Vitamin $B_{12}$.

12 True – in this double-blind study, 59% of patients maintained their remission for 1 year on fish oil capsules, and 26% on placebo capsules.

13 a 40–60 mg once daily for 4 weeks.

b 15%.

c Azathioprine.

14 a False – it is rare in infants, probably because there are no receptors for the toxin.

b False – it usually presents as a watery diarrhoea.

c False – it is best treated with metronidazole or vancomycin.

15 Since 19% of colonic cancers are due to familial polyposis and 5–15% are due to non-adenomatous cancer with an autosomal inheritance, ideally one could find out whether other relatives had a similar problem, at what age the patient's father developed the cancer, and whether the father had adenomas before the final illness, but this may be impossible.

The risk of colonic cancer is lower in individuals with a low intake of meat, and patients may be told of this. The balance of evidence suggests that regular prophylaxis with aspirin reduces the risk of colonic cancer. Since it also reduces the risk of vascular disease, those at increased risk of colonic cancer should be encouraged to use it.

One may advise the patient to bring any abdominal symptoms or suspicion of anaemia to medical attention at an early stage. Screening with FOBs detects about 60% of colonic cancers before they cause symptoms, but the general population complies poorly with this measure, although those with a family history may give it more priority. If the father's cancer was known to be preceded by multiple adenomas, the offspring should undergo colonoscopy. Gene mapping will probably also have a role when it is available.

16  Sedentary workers have readier access to a toilet, and so may more easily respond to a sense of rectal fullness.

17  a  Most experts consider that those with a family history of colonic cancer in two or more first-degree relatives should be screened from the age of 25 years. Those with a history of colonic cancer in one first-degree relative should be screened after the age of 40 years, especially if the cancer occurred before the age of 55 years, as they have a 1.7-fold risk of the disease.

   b  Recommended guidelines for screening subjects with hereditary non-polyposis colorectal cancer syndrome (i.e. colorectal cancer in at least three family members spanning two generations, with one or more cases diagnosed before the age of 50 years) are as follows:
   • colonoscopy from the age of 20–25 years every 2 years
   • gastroscopy from the age of 35 years every 1–2 years
   • urinary ultrasound and cytology from the age of 30–35 years every 1–2 years for associated bladder or renal cancer
   • for associated ovarian cancer, transvaginal ultrasound and assay of CA-125 from the age of 30 years every 1–2 years.

   c  2%.

   d  i  1.0–9.8%.
      ii  8–17%, typically 20–30% in the screened group and 9–22% in controls.
      iii  15–33%.
      iv  53–75%.

   e  Red and white meat, fish, raw vegetables and fruits containing peroxidase should be avoided.

   f  80%.

18  a  True.
    b  False – only 2 of 10 cases in this study.
    c  False – only about 25% returned them.

19  a  9.
    b  12.

20  20%.

21  a  False – the true figure is up to 7%.

   b  False – in this series, 7 of 89 patients would have had a diagnosis of colonic cancer missed if the upper gastrointestinal tract only had been investigated.

   c  True – up to 50% of colonoscopies by inexperienced operators fail to reach the caecum.

22  False – anaemia and weight loss are more likely presentations.

23  Most doctors answering this question mentioned that those patients with associated perianal pain or an obvious haemorrhoid or fissure could be investigated and treated first in the GP surgery. Others might also be investigated by DRE and proctoscopy by the GP, but if no cause was found they would probably require referral for further investigation. A single episode of unexplained bleeding would justify referral if the patient was over 40 years old, or in younger patients with a family history of polyposis or carcinoma of the rectum, or if there were associated findings of iron deficiency anaemia, altered bowel habit, weight loss or systemic upset. Unexplained recurrent bleeding always justifies referral.

24  Every 3–5 years.

25  Carcinoembryonic antigen.

26  The bowel preparation treatment will cause you to have diarrhoea which may make you dehydrated. Drink one or two cups or glasses of fluid after every loose bowel movement.

27  Proctalgia fugax.

28  Insert a gloved and lubricated finger to stretch the puborectalis muscle.

29  a  False.

   b  True.

30  It relaxes the anal sphincter, thus improving blood flow.

# HAEMATOLOGY

**1** Iron deficiency. (*True/False*)

   **a** Middle-aged women are particularly subject to oesophageal and pharyngeal webs.

   **b** A normal serum ferritin level may coexist with iron deficiency in the presence of an inflammatory disorder.

   **c** Cow's milk contains more iron than formula milk.

*BMJ.* **314**: 360–3 (review)

**2** Anaemia in the elderly.

   **a** What is the lower limit of normal for the haemoglobin level in an elderly person?

   **b** How large are red cells likely to be in a patient with myelodysplasia?

   **c** How might you investigate an elderly patient with Hb 95 g/L and mean cell volume (MCV) 84 fL?

*BMJ.* **314**: 1262–5 (review)

**3** Macrocytosis. (*True/False*)

   **a** Two gin and tonics a day are enough to raise the mean cell volume of the erythrocytes above 100 fL.

   **b** Intrinsic factor antibodies are present in all cases of pernicious anaemia.

   **c** Initial treatment of pernicious anaemia is with an injection of 1 mg of hydroxycobalamin every 3 months.

   **d** A mother who has had a baby with a neural tube defect should take 400 mg of folate daily before and during subsequent pregnancies.

*BMJ.* **314**: 430–3 (review)

**4** An elderly patient has a macrocytic anaemia and a low serum vitamin $B_{12}$ level. What further investigations will you arrange?

*BMJ.* **304**: 1584–5

**5** You come across a patient who has been receiving regular injections of vitamin $B_{12}$ for no reason that you can discern from her history or notes. How will you go about determining whether she is deriving any benefit from these injections? (*2 or more points*)

BMJ. **311**: 28–30

**6** Blood donation.

a What is the usual minimum recommended period between blood dona- tions in the UK?

b What event is liable to occur even in experienced regular donors in the 24 h after donation?

BMJ. **314**: 863 (question and answer)

**7** Warfarin.

a What is its elimination half-life?

b What is a suitable loading dose for Chinese people?

BMJ. **313**: 301–2 (letter)

**8** Variation in intake of what dietary constituent is likely to affect the warfarin requirement for anticoagulation?

BMJ. **314**: 1386 (research report)

**9** What form of infection appears to be a particular danger to people with chronic lymphoproliferative malignancies, including multiple myeloma? (*1 point*)

BMJ. **311**: 26–7

**10** What clinical features in patients treated for Hodgkin's disease are suffi- ciently likely to indicate relapse as to justify forewarning the patient? (*4 or more points*)

BMJ. **314**: 343–6 (research report)

**11** Hyposplenism.

a What features on a full blood count suggest this diagnosis? (*4 points*)

b What conditions may cause functional hyposplenism? (*9 points*)

c What should be done to prevent patients with hyposplenism from suffering infections? (*6 points*)

BMJ. **312**: 430–3 (guideline article)

**12** Polycythaemia.

**a** What should be done to check that a raised packed cell volume (PCV) is not due to an artefact of sampling?

**b** What are the possible presenting features of primary polycythaemia?

**c** What bedside observation will differentiate primary from secondary polycythaemia?

**d** What target PCV is suggested for patients with:

  i  primary polycythaemia

  ii  polycythaemia secondary to hypoxia

  iii  polycythaemia secondary to renal disease

  iv  apparent polycythaemia (raised PCV but normal red cell mass)?

**e** What are the clinical features of idiopathic myelofibrosis?

*BMJ.* **314**: 587–60 (review)

**13**   What are the clinical features of idiopathic myelofibrosis?

*BMJ.* **314**: 587–60 (review)

**14**   Myelodysplasia.

**a** What are the common presenting clinical features?

**b** What is the prognosis?

**c** What treatment options are available?

*BMJ.* **314**: 883–6 (review)

**15**   Myeloma.

**a** What are the clinical features associated with hyperviscosity syndrome? (*4 points*)

**b** What percentage of cases have a high ESR? (*1 point*)

**c** What treatments may help the associated hypercalcaemia found in 30% of cases? (*3 points*)

**d** What is the prognosis for someone with a monoclonal gammopathy of undetermined significance? (*2 points*)

*BMJ.* **314**: 960–3 (review)

**16**   After a marrow transplant:

**a** what viral infections are prevalent while patients are immunosuppressed? (*3 points*)

**b** what fungal infections are prevalent while patients are immunosuppressed? (*2 points*)

**c** what are the presenting features of acute graft-vs.-host disease? (*4 points*)

**d** what are the presenting features of chronic graft-vs.-host disease? (*8 points*)

*BMJ.* **314**: 1179–82 (review)

**17** Coagulation disorders.

**a** Which clinical features of a bleeding disorder suggest a coagulation defect, and which suggest a platelet defect? (*8 points*)

**b** What proportion of patients with venous thrombosis have an inherited condition causing thrombophilia?

**c** What circumstances make testing for antithrombin, protein S and protein C unreliable? (*2 points*)

*BMJ.* **314**: 1026–9 (review)

**18** Hereditary anaemias. (*True/False*)

**a** Sickle cell anaemia is restricted to Africans.

**b** Aspirin causes haemolysis in men with glucose-6-phosphate dehydrogenase deficiency.

*BMJ.* **314**: 492–6 (review)

**19** Sickle cell disease.

**a** At what stage in reproductive life is it most appropriate to screen for haemoglobinopathies?

**b** What regime of antipneumococcal vaccine is appropriate for sufferers?

**c** What infection is the main cause of hypoplastic crises?

**d** How prevalent is bone pain in sufferers?

**e** What home treatment is appropriate for bone pain?

**f** What other complications of the condition may present as emergencies? (*10 points*)

**g** What regime of penicillin is appropriate for children aged:

   i under 12 months

   ii 1–3 years

   iii over 3 years?

**h** What circumstances are liable to provoke crises?

**i** What physical examination technique may usefully be demonstrated to parents?

**j** Why is smoking particularly to be avoided?

**k** What vitamin supplement may be useful?

**l** What emergency treatment is required for splenic sequestration?

**m** What emergency treatment is required for an acute chest syndrome?

**n** What procedure offers a good prospect of cure if sufferers are in reasonable health?

**o** What form of haemoglobin interferes with the sickling process in sickle cell anaemia and is increased by treatment with hydroxyurea?

**p** What are the benefits and dangers of hydroxyurea treatment?

*BMJ.* **315**: 656–60 (review)

*BMJ.* **310**: 352

**20** What are the common causes of death in patients with sickle cell disease? (*5 points*). For each of these list one or more preventive techniques. (*5 points*)

*BMJ.* **311**: 1600–1 (research report)

**21** A successful liver transplant will cure haemophilia. (*True/False*)

*BMJ.* **316**: 1684 (citation)

# ANSWERS

1   a  True.

    b  True – or in the presence of liver disease.

    c  False.

2   a  110 g/L.

    b  Normocytic or macrocytic.

    c  The author's suggestion, in order of priority, is as follows: review film for evidence of marrow disorder, ferritin, vitamin $B_{12}$ and folate levels, urinalysis, ESR, LFT, U&E, CXR, autoantibody screen, thyroid function test, and finally as tumour markers, gamma-globulin electrophoresis, prostate-specific antigen, alpha-fetoprotein and carcinoembryonic antigen.

3   a  True.

    b  False – they are present in 50% of cases and parietal cell antibodies are present in 90% of cases.

    c  False – six injections of 1 mg of hydroxycobalamin should be given at intervals of 3–4 days. Injections should then be given every 3 months.

    d  False – in this high-risk group the appropriate daily dose is 5 mg.

4   A combination of macrocytic anaemia and a low serum vitamin $B_{12}$ may be due to dietary deficiency, intestinal malabsorption, pernicious anaemia or possibly a laboratory artefact or spuriously low level of serum vitamin $B_{12}$, since this last measurement is quite labile. A dietary history, questions about bowel habit and any alteration in weight may rule out the first two causes. Repeating the vitamin $B_{12}$ assay may be simpler than bone-marrow examination to confirm the deficiency. Intrinsic factor antibodies may then confirm that true pernicious anaemia is present. If not, a Schilling test would be advisable before the patient is committed to a lifetime of $B_{12}$ injections. If the diagnosis is confirmed, thyroid function tests and gastroscopy may or may not be clinically indicated. However, good note-taking is required if future doctors seeing the patient are to be aware of the justification for treatment.

5   Several doctors answering this question suggested delaying the patient's next appointment for 3 months, and then sending off for a full blood count and vitamin $B_{12}$ level. Those with normal results would then have this procedure repeated every 2 months thereafter for 6 months.

6   a  12 weeks, but usually only two donations per year are allowed.

    b  Fainting.

7   a  35 h.

    b  5 mg/day for 2 days.

8   Vitamin K in green vegetables.

9 Pneumococcal septicaemia.

10 The author suggests lump, cough, night sweats and weight loss. Consider also alcohol-induced pain, itch, lethargy, dyspnoea, rash and reduced appetite.

11 a Howell-Jolly bodies, Heinz bodies, thrombocytosis and monocytosis.
   b Sickle cell anaemia, thalassaemia major, essential thrombocythaemia, lymphoma, chronic lymphocytic leukaemia, coeliac disease, dermatitis herpetiformis, inflammatory bowel disease and bone marrow transplant.
   c • Pneumococcal vaccine every 5–10 years.
     • Flu vaccine annually.
     • *Haemophilus influenzae* type B vaccine.
     • Mengivac if travelling to areas where types A and C may cause infection.
     • Ensure that the patient takes particular care to avoid malaria.
     • Penicillin or amoxycillin or erythromycin daily for life.
     • A supply of amoxycillin for home use if a feverish illness supervenes or if the patient suffers a bite.
     • Provide an information booklet or card that the patient can carry around with details of these precautions.

12 a Take a blood sample without occlusion.
   b Stroke, TIA, ischaemic digits, headache, mental clouding, facial redness, itching, abnormal bleeding and gout.
   c The presence of splenomegaly.
   d  i 0.45.
      ii 0.50–0.52.
      iii 0.45.
      iv 0.54.

13 Splenomegaly, weight loss, anaemia, fatigue and bleeding.

14 a Anaemia, infection due to neutropenia, and bleeding due to thrombocytopenia.
   b Median survival 20 months, with death due to marrow failure or leukaemic change.
   c Observation, transfusion, antibiotics, haemopoietic growth factors, chemotherapy, differentiating agents, or bone marrow transplant.

15 a Impaired CNS functions, impaired vision, purpura, haemorrhage.
   b 10%.
   c Rehydration, diuresis and, if necessary, biphosphonate.
   d Multiple myeloma, macroglobulinaemia, amyloidosis or lymphoma ultimately develop in 26% of cases, with an actuarial rate of 16% at 10 years.

16 a Herpes zoster, herpes simplex and cytomegalovirus pneumonia.
   b Candida and aspergillus.
   c Abdominal pain, diarrhoea, jaundice, and skin rash on palms and soles.

**d** Dry skin, dry eyes and mouth, mucosal ulcers, malabsorption, recurrent chest infections, cholestatic jaundice, restricted joint movements, pneumococcal infection due to hyposplenism and myelosuppression.

17  **a** Coagulation defects are commonly associated with bleeding into the tissues, such as bruises, haemarthrosis and haematuria, and dental bleeding delayed for 12–24 h after treatment, whereas platelet disorders are associated with external bleeding such as profuse bleeding from cuts, nosebleeds, gastrointestinal bleeding, and bleeding immediately after dentistry.

   **b** 50%.

   **c** The presence of an active thrombus, and current use of anticoagulants.

18  **a** False – it is also found in the Mediterranean countries, the Middle East and parts of India.

   **b** True – and so do phenacetin, primaquine, pamaquine, sulphonamides, nalidixic acid and dapsone.

19  **a** Before conception.

   **b** A half dose at 10–12 months, than a full dose at 3 years and every 3 to 5 years thereafter.

   **c** Human parvovirus B19.

   **d** It is experienced on up to 30% of days, with a loss of 10% of schooldays in children.

   **e** Increased fluid intake, rest, warmth, massage, simple analgesics (including NSAIDs, but avoiding opiates stronger than codeine).

   **f** Swollen painful joints, CNS deficit, acute sickle chest syndrome or pneumonia, mesenteric sickling and bowel ischaemia, splenic or hepatic sequestration, cholecystitis, renal papillary necrosis resulting in colic or haematuria, priapism, hyphaema and retinal detachment.

   **g** Penicillin dose for prophylaxis:

      i 62.5 mg once or twice daily

     ii 125 mg daily

    iii 250 mg daily.

   **h** Cold, dehydration, exhaustion, and prolonged or severe infection.

   **i** How to examine for splenic or hepatic enlargement.

   **j** It may provide chest crises.

   **k** Folic acid.

   **l** Blood transfusion.

   **m** Oxygen, continuous positive airways pressure, and exchange transfusion.

   **n** Marrow transplant.

   **o** Fetal haemoglobin.

   **p** • Benefits – fewer painful crises, and lower incidence of chest syndrome.
   - Dangers – its myelosuppressive and teratogenic effects necessitate caution, its long-term toxicity appears to be low but is not yet well qualified, and it may

transform chronic leukaemia and myeloproliferative disorders into acute leukaemia.

**20** All the common causes of death are less common if the patient attends a specialist clinic and is made aware of the need for prompt treatment of any complication. In addition, bone marrow transplantation and hydroxyurea treatment reduce the incidence of thrombotic and aplastic complications.

- Acute splenic sequestration – education of patients and parents, prophylactic splenectomy after two or more episodes, oxygen.
- Acute chest syndrome – transfusion.
- Septicaemia-meningitis – prophylactic penicillin, pneumococcal and haemophilus vaccination.
- Stroke – transfusion may reduce the rate of recurrence.
- Aplastic crisis – early hospitalization, transfusion and oxygen, parvovirus vaccine.
- Portal vein thrombosis.

**21** True.

# HUMAN IMMUNODEFICIENCY DISEASE

## Testing

**1** Testing for HIV antibodies.

    **a** What screening test is sensitive but not specific?

    **b** What confirmatory test, when combined with two screening tests, is 99% accurate?

*BMJ.* **316**: 1039 (news item)

**2** Women in the UK who are HIV-positive.

    **a** What proportion of the HIV-positive population in the UK do they constitute?

    **b** What proportion of those who are HIV-positive are aware of it?

    **b** What proportion are registered with a GP?

    **c** Of those registered with a GP and who are aware of their condition, what proportion have told their GP of it?

*Br J Gen Pract.* **48**: 1329–30 (survey report)

**3** Human immunodeficiency virus.

    **a** What proportion of babies in London are born to mothers who are HIV-positive?

    **b** What is the current best estimate of the reduction in risk of HIV in the infant if mothers who are HIV-positive are made aware of this in early pregnancy?

*BMJ.* **316**: 1333 (research report)

**4** Why may it be particularly advantageous to test women for HIV when they have a termination of a pregnancy?

*BMJ.* **316**: 1899 (letter)

**5** What can be done to minimize the impact on a marriage of discovering that one partner is HIV-positive? (*3 or more points*)

*BMJ.* **311**:1578 (personal statement)

**6** What would be the advantages and disadvantages of patients being able to test themselves for HIV antibodies with home kits? (*4 or more points*)

*BMJ.* **313**: 1354 (news item)

# Symptoms and signs

**1** What skin condition affects the majority of patients affected with HIV and is recognized as an indicator in stage II of the disease? (*1 point*)

*BMJ.* **311**:1514 (citation)

**2** HIV infection. (*10 points*)

**a** What are the clinical features of the acute retroviral seroconversion syndrome which initially affects 30–60% of people who contract HIV infection?

**b** What blood assays are most likely to confirm the diagnosis at this stage?

*BMJ.* **314**: 487–91 (review)

# Management

**1** What efforts should we make to prevent HIV-positive patients from cross-infecting each other?

*BMJ.* **315**: 1317 (view)

**2** What would be appropriate investigations and management for the following symptoms in a patient with AIDS?

**a** Cough. (*4 points*)

**b** Anorexia, nausea, vomiting. (*4 points*)

**c** Retrosternal pain. (*3 points*)

**d** Chronic severe headache. (*3 points*)

**e** Abdominal pain. (*4 points*)

**f**  Perineal pain. (*4 points*)

*BMJ.* **315**: 1433–6 (review)

**3**  Two homosexual men who are HIV-positive can have unprotected inter-course with each other with impunity. (*True/False)*

*BMJ.* **316**: 84 (citation)

**4**  What combination of treatment is reported to limit transmission of HIV to the infants of infected pregnant mothers to 1%?

*BMJ.* **317**: 11 (news item)

# ANSWERS

## Testing

1   a Enzyme-linked immunosorbent assay (ELISA).
    b Western blot.

2   a 15%.
    b 13%.
    c 81%.
    d 83%.

3   a 1 in 520.
    b The use of antiretroviral drugs in pregnancy reduces transmission by two-thirds. Further reductions can be made by Caesarean section and by advising the mother not to breast-feed.

4   Young single women are the fastest growing group of new cases of HIV infection. Identifying them and informing them of the diagnosis at the time of a termination may make them reconsider whether to have a further pregnancy, and may ensure that they receive appropriate treatment.

5   The article which drew our attention to this problem was based on African society, but problems in a Western marriage are scarcely less severe if one partner is found to be HIV-positive. The matter needs to be discussed before any test is arranged. The patient needs to be warned of the possibility that the partner may leave the relationship. Ideally, any infidelities would be discussed between the partners before the test proceeds. The partners can then be counselled together on prognosis and precautions while the disaster is still hypothetical, and after allowing time for the implications to sink in both partners can then be tested. However, if this cannot be achieved the suspect should still be tested.

    If faced with a positive result, the patient needs to be told first and encouraged to reattend with their partner for a fuller discussion. Ready access to the doctor and to support groups should be provided to both parties while they come to terms with the loss of previous expectations.

6   Anonymous self-testing for HIV is now possible in America as a sampling kit has been marketed, and the blot of blood is despatched to a central laboratory. Proponents argue that the use of such kits will increase the uptake of tests, is less expensive than conventional testing, and that 85% of users listen to the information tape which is provided with the kit. For the individual whose test proves positive, it permits him or her to remain discreet about how he or she uses the information, thus perhaps preserving a marriage, or allowing for purchase of a family home.

Anxieties about the service centre on the lack of assurance that users have received advice about lifestyle implications, support arrangements and treatment if the test proves positive, lack of assurance that users understand that the test may not become positive for up to 9 months after exposure, the possibility of poor technique leading to inaccurate results, blackmail, and the inability to obtain epidemiological information if many patients undergo tests but fail to reveal their results.

# Symptoms and signs

1   Seborrhoeic dermatitis.

2   a   Fever, myalgia, maculopapular rash, lymphadenopathy and, less commonly, oral ulcers, neurological manifestations and occasionally markers of immuno-suppression such as oral candidiasis, acute leucopenia and an acute reduction in CD4 lymphocytes.

   b   Viral p24 antigen in serum or HIV RNA in plasma-resistant strain.

# Management

1   Advise these patients on handwashing and maintaining cleanliness with regard to the bathroom, clothing and cooking. Advise them to consult immediately if they develop respiratory symptoms, and obtain X-rays and sputum samples early for TB. Some cross-infection occurs at clinics, so sputum samples should be obtained while the patient is alone. If there is a significant risk of TB these patients should be isolated.

2   a   Cough – sputum sample, TB cultures, chest X-ray (to exclude *Pneumocystis carinii* and Kaposi's sarcoma).

   b   Anorexia, nausea, vomiting – enquire about constipation, check for drug side-effects, mouth swab for candida, scans or endoscopy for tumours.

   c   Retrosternal pain – endoscopy and swabs for candida cytomegalovirus and herpes simplex, and chest X-ray for *Pneumcystis carinii*.

   d   Chronic severe headache – lumbar puncture for protein, sugar, cells, toxoplasma, cryptococcus, CT or MMR scan for lymphoma.

   e   Abdominal pain – check bowel habit, ultrasound for sclerosing cholangitis, arrange endoscopy and ultrasound for tumour.

   f   Perineal pain – check and swab for herpes simplex and candida, barrier cream for excoriation from diarrhoea.

3    False – they may not be infected by the same strain, and one may be infected with a drug-resistant strain.

4    Zidovudine and a Caesarean section.

# INFECTION

## Prevention

**1** What proportion of patients who are admitted to hospital acquire an infection?

*BMJ.* **315**: 1315–16 (personal view)

**2** Patients on long-term oral steroids should be warned of the risk of chickenpox. How should the warning be worded? (*3 points*)

*BMJ.* **312**:: 542–3 (research report)

**3** During a flu epidemic the following categories of patient should take amantadine: (*True/False*)

**a** a child with catarrh and diarrhoea

**b** the unvaccinated residents of a block of warden-controlled flats where one resident has symptoms of flu

**c** an unvaccinated patient who is HIV-positive

**d** an unvaccinated resident in a nursing home who develops catarrh, myalgia and fever

**e** an unvaccinated GP

**f** an unvaccinated asthmatic on oral steroids.

*BMJ.* **302**: 425–6

**4** What infection may be spread by birds pecking milk-bottle tops on doorsteps?

*BMJ.* **303**: 1560

**5** What hygiene measure particularly needs to be promoted to doctors to prevent the spread of methicillin-resistant *Staphylococcus aureus*?

*BMJ.* **315**: 59 (correspondence)

**6** List three or more diseases that may justify the intervention of public health authorities even though they are not currently notifiable?

*BMJ.* **304**: 726–7, 755, 1056

**7** With which organisms are patients who have undergone splenectomy particularly susceptible to infection? (*4 points*)

*BMJ.* **312**: 1360 (letter)

**8** A splenectomized patient: (*True/False*)

**a** requires only one dose of pneumococcal vaccine

**b** requires 250 mg penicillin V twice daily for life.

*BMJ.* **307**: 1372–3

**9** What chemoprophylaxis should be offered to family members of a child with epiglottitis due to *Haemophilus influenzae* Type B, who has a sibling under 3 years of age?

*BMJ.* **302**: 546–7

# Diagnosis

**1** How long does a thermometer placed in the axilla take to equilibrate?

*BMJ.* **304**: 931–2

**2** Lyme disease. (*True/False*)

**a** The rash may be confused with that of ringworm.

**b** Antibody tests are likely to be positive within 2 weeks of infection.

**c** Erythromycin is a recommended treatment.

*BMJ.* **310**: 303–8

# Respiratory and upper respiratory tract infection

**1** The following appear to be associated with an increased probability of culturing group A streptococci from a sore throat: (*True/False*)

**a** season – October to December

**b** the patient being a young child

**c** duration of less than 3 days

**d** bad smell

**e** sore ears

**f** cough

**g** abdominal pain

**h** vomiting

**i** fever

**j** muscle aches

**k** headache

**l** swollen glands in the anterior triangle

**m** exudate on the tonsils.

*Br J Gen Pract.* **41**: 504–7

*Br J Gen Pract.* **46**: 4614 (research reports)

**2** An adult with a sore throat which swab culture subsequently shows to be harbouring group B haemolytic streptococci is prescribed penicillin. What benefits can be expected from the treatment? (*2 points*)

*Br J Gen Pract.* **46**: 589–93

**3** What carriage rate for beta-haemolytic streptococci can be expected:

**a** in the healthy population

**b** in patients with URTIs?

*BMJ.* **311**: 193

**4** What organisms are associated with pneumonia accompanied by the following clinical features?

**a** Sore throat, nausea, diarrhoea, chills and myalgia.

**b** Severe pneumonia during a flu epidemic.

*BMJ.* **308**: 701–4

# Gastrointestinal infection

**1** When managing a patient with diarrhoea which started within the past week, how would the following observations influence your further investigations or treatment?

**a** Stools, although frequent, are of small volume.

**b** The patient is a promiscuous homosexual.

**c** The patient has eaten reheated rice within the past 6 h.

**d** Th patient developed diarrhoea while on holiday in Spain, and returned to the UK yesterday.

**e** The onset of watery diarrhoea occurred 5 days ago, and blood in the stools 3 days ago.

**f** The patient is feverish.

**g** The patient is dizzy on standing.

*BMJ.* **304**: 1302–5

**2** A temporary resident at a local hotel has gastroenteritis and thinks that he may make a claim on his holiday insurance. What can you as the GP who sees him suggest be done in order that the claim can be evaluated? (*2 or more points*)

*BMJ.* **312**: 925–6 (leading article)

**3** If people aged over 45 years take omeprazole, to what infection will they be particularly susceptible in the following month?

*BMJ.* **312**: 414–15 (research report)

**4** Which vitamin, and at what dose, has been found to accelerate resolution of symptoms in malnourished children treated with antibiotics for shigella dysentery, although it has no effect on bacteriological clearance?

*BMJ.* **316**: 422–5 (research report)

**5** Chronic amoebiasis can be diagnosed by serology. (*True/False*)

*BMJ.* **309**: 490

# Skin and soft tissue infections

**1** Where would you obtain tetanus immune globulin to give to a patient with a dirty, infected wound who has not had tetanus toxoid in the last 10 years?

*Br J Gen Pract.* **41**: 41

**2** Prescription of which vitamin, and at what dose, is likely to reduce the complication rate in measles according to the results of studies from the UK and Africa?

*BMJ.* **301**: 1230

**3** Which infections can cause a vaginal itch?

*BMJ.* **304**: 1648

**4** For which patients with herpes zoster is acyclovir or famciclovir treatment justified? (*3 points*)

*Br J Gen Pract.* **45**: 3945 (review)

**5** What advice would you give to an elderly patient with localized herpes zoster on prevention and control of post-herpetic neuralgia?

*Br J Gen Pract.* **305**: 244–6

**6** For which patients with chickenpox is treatment with acyclovir indicated? (*2 points*)

*BMJ.* **310**: 108–10 (discussion papers)

**7** Roseola infantum: (*True/False*)

**a** mainly affects infants aged 2 – 4 years

**b** mainly affects the face

**c** causes a lacy rash.

*BMJ.* **312**: 101–2

**8** What are the clinical features of scarlatina? (*4 points*)

*BMJ.* **315**: 1492 (anecdote)

**9** What tests are appropriate for establishing the diagnosis when fluid is withdrawn from what appears to be a septic bursa?

*BMJ.* **316**: 1877 (research report)

# Meningitis

**1** What is the second most commonest form of rash seen in children with meningococcal disease? (*1 point*)

*BMJ.* **313**: 1255–6 (case reports)

**2** If meningitis causes cerebral irritation, how may it present?

*BMJ.* **306**: 775–6

**3** What sample(s) might a GP take to enable a laboratory to reach a positive diagnosis of meningococcal septicaemia? (*2 points*)

*BMJ.* **314**:831–2 (correspondence)

*BMJ.* **306**: 775–6

**4** **a** In what proportion of cases of systemic meningococcal infection can the bacterium be isolated from a swab of the posterior pharyngeal wall?

**b** Why may it be useful to take a sequestrene sample early in a case of bacterial meningitis?

*BMJ.* **315**: 757–8 (leading article)

**5** You have injected penicillin and despatched a 6-year-old child to hospital with fever, lethargy, a stiff neck and a petechial rash. What will you do for his parents and for his sister aged 6 months? (*3 or more points*)

*Br J Gen Pract.* **47**: 201–2

**6** Apart from penicillin, what other anti-infective agents may be of benefit for emergency treatment of a child with meningitis without a microbiological diagnosis? (*1 point*)

*BMJ.* **304**: 116

*BMJ.* **310**: 139–40 (editorial)

# ANSWERS

## Prevention

1 About 10%.

2 If you have not had chickenpox, avoid contact with any person who has chickenpox or shingles, and if you have been exposed to chickenpox or shingles, seek urgent medical attention.

3 a False – diarrhoea suggests an infection other than flu.

 b True – amantadine confers about 50% protection, and results in a milder illness in 70–100% of the remaining cases.

 c True –they are immunocompromised.

 d False – giving amantadine might encourage the development of a resistant strain.

 e True – this worker is at particular risk.

 f True – they are immunocompromised and the after-effects might be long-lasting.

4 *Campylobacter* enteric infection.

5 Handwashing.

6 The authors suggest Lyme disease, Legionnaire's disease, toxoplasmosis, listeriosis, toxocariasis and cryptosporidiosis.

7 *Pneumococcus*, *Meningococcus*, malarial parasites, *Haemophilus influenzae*, tick-borne organisms.

8 a False.

 b True.

9 Rifampicin – 20 mg/kg up to 600 mg/day for 4 days.

## Diagnosis

1 9 min.

2 a True.

 b False – this requires several weeks.

 c False.

## Respiratory and upper respiratory tract infection

1  a True.
   b True.
   c True.
   d True.
   e False.
   f False.
   g False.
   h False.
   i True.
   j True.
   k False
   l True.
   m True.

2  Duration of pain reduced by 1 to 2 days, and shorter duration of fever.

3  a 0.6%.
   b 9.6%.

4  a *Mycoplasma.*
   b *Staphylococcus.*

## Gastrointestinal infection

1  a Probable irritable bowel syndrome – consider antispasmodics.
   b Possible *Giardia lambda* infection.
   c Possible *Bacillus cereus* infection – stool culture required.
   d Probable *E. coli* – consider trimethoprim treatment.
   e Possible shigella dysentery – send off stool sample and consider giving ampicillin.
   f Suggests shigella or campylobacter infection or dehydration – consider stool culture, blood culture and parenteral fluids.
   g Suggests dehydration – consider the possibility that intravenous fluids may be needed.

2  • A history of all food and drink ingested during the 3 days before symptoms started, from the patient and from all members of his party.

- Stools for microbiology from the patient to be sent to the environmental health laboratory.
- The hotelier to be informed of the problem, and the doctor to suggest that any remaining suspect food be sent for microbiological examination by the environmental health laboratory.
- The doctor to give the guest his address and telephone number and to offer to provide a report to the insurer or tour operator.

3 Campylobacter enteritis – the incidence is increased by 10- to 12-fold. Although the incidence is still quite low, the authors comment that patients with diarrhoea who are taking omeprazole should have a faecal culture.

4 Vitamin A – 200 000 IU as a single dose.

5 True.

# Skin and soft tissue infections

1 Blood transfusion service.

2 Vitamin A – 400 000 IU irrespective of age.

3 Trichomonas, herpes, thrush, warts, lice and threadworms.

4 Patients who are elderly, in pain, or who have a rash affecting the upper face.

5 The author suggests advising the patient to come back if burning pain is a problem, as early treatment (with amitriptyline) may make a difference.

6 Those who are immunocompromised and adults with onset of chickenpox within the previous 24 h.

7 a False – it mainly affects infants aged 40–60 weeks.
 b False – it mainly affects the thighs and buttocks.
 c False – it usually causes macules with a surrounding halo.

8 Strawberry tongue, fine generalized exfoliating erythematous rash, nappy rash and fever.

9 Culture in a liquid medium. Staphylococci are the commonest organism cultured. Cytological examination, particularly for neutrophils.

# Meningitis

1   Maculopapular.

2   Agitation, violence, as well as stupor or coma.

3   Throat swab, sequestrene sample, scrape a skin lesion and spread blood on a glass slide for microscopy. Blood culture if bottles are available.

4   a  About half.

    b  Polymerase chain reaction on such a scrape may reveal bacterial antigen even when blood culture is negative.

5   For the parents, chemoprophylaxis should be with rifampicin 600 mg twice daily for 2 days. For the baby, rifampicin 5 mg/kg bd for 2 days or ceftriaxone 125 mg i.m. Remind parents to be vigilant for rash or fever and to seek medical advice immediately if they develop. Consider giving Mengivac AC if A or C strains are prevalent in the area.

6   Chloramphenicol injection if the patient is allergic to penicillin. Intravenous acyclovir if possibly due to herpetic meningitis.

# MEDICINE FOR THE ELDERLY

**1** Which symptoms might usefully be brought to the attention of elderly people as justifying mentioning to their GPs?

*Br J Gen Pract.* **47**: 427–30 (research report)

**2** On a home visit you find an 80-year-old woman in an untidy house wearing stained clothes. She has not been seen by a doctor for several months. With difficulty, due to her limited hearing and her dementia, you obtain a history of watery diarrhoea for 'some time' and observe her leg oedema, her varicose eczema and her fruity cough. She is breathless when walking about the house. She has a supply of a loop diuretic and vitamin pills and appears to use these erratically. She lives alone, and a home help comes three times a week to do her shopping and housework. She has no relatives in the vicinity. You decide to refer her to the local consultant geriatrician. What considerations will affect your decision on whether you ask for her to be admitted, seen at out-patients urgently or seen at a domiciliary visit?

*BMJ.* **302**: 426–71, 655–6

**3** An old lady who lives alone has fallen out of bed at 5 a.m. and rung her telephone alert. What do you need to assess in order to determine whether she can stay at home on her own:

**a** within an hour

**b** within a day?

*BMJ.* **316**: 1174 (anecdote)

**4** You find yourself at loggerheads with the carer of an elderly woman with unexplained symptoms which you ascribe to depression and which the carer ascribes to a physical cause. The patient herself is rather apathetic about the matter. What are the advantages and disadvantages of obtaining a second opinion? What alternatives are there to resolving the situation to the patient's advantage?

*BMJ.* **311**: 670–2 (opinion statements)

**5** What provision is there for night-sitting highly dependent patients at home, and how can such a service be financed, other than by the patient or their family?

*BMJ.* **307**:915–18

**6** Should GPs be active in putting active, willing pensioners in contact with ill or housebound pensioners in the same locality to help them with their problems? State reasons for your point of view.

*Br J Gen Pract.* **41**: 382–5

**7** Taking part in an exercise programme has been associated with a reduced rate of falls in elderly women. What types of exercises appear to be practical and helpful?

*BMJ.* **314**: 569 (trial report)

**8** What misfortune may befall an elderly person just after eating a large meal rich in carbohydrate?

*BMJ.* **308**: 730

**9** Paget's disease.

  **a** What other conditions does the pain produced mimic?

  **b** What routine biochemical tests are useful if screening for the condition?

  **c** For how long should oral biphosphonate treatment be continued?

  **d** What monitoring is useful thereafter?

*BMJ.* **312**: 491–4 (review)

**10** Treating asymptomatic bacteriuria is likely to cure incontinence in the elderly. (*True/False*)

*BMJ.* **310**: 1616

**11** A patient whose only complaint is nocturia may benefit from the following: (*True/False*)

  **a** increasing fluid intake if it has been restricted

  **b** substituting bland fluids for coffee.

*BMJ.* **307**: 1354

**12** 'I feel dizzy if I walk out of doors.' The elderly lady who made this statement is housebound as a result, but has no other disabilities or psychological problems, no other symptoms or signs to suggest heart failure, and the only finding on examination is dizziness on extreme neck movements, especially when erect. How might you help her?

*BMJ.* **308**: 1252–3

**13** A patient who is dissatisfied with his hearing when using an NHS hearing aid may benefit from a privately fitted implantable hearing aid. (*True/False*)

*BMJ.* **309**: 651–4

**14** Quinine. (*True/False*)

**a** It probably reduces the frequency of night cramps by about 30%.

**b** It greatly reduces the severity of night cramps.

**c** The benefits on night cramps are apparent from the first night of taking the drug.

**d** It may cause pancytopenia.

*BMJ.* **310**: 13–16 (research report)

**15** What drug in addition to quinine has been shown to be effective in treating night cramps?

*BMJ.* **310**: 1138

**16** 'When I turn my car to the left I feel a sort of grating in my back.' This complaint sounds musculoskeletal in nature, but what else might it be?

*BMJ.* **316**: 786 (anecdote)

# ANSWERS

1 Judging from the data in the report, treatable symptoms that elderly people are unlikely to bring to medical attention include fluttering in the chest, tightness in the chest on walking uphill, breathlessness, tiredness and low spirits. Members also suggested fatigue, polyuria, altered bowel habit and light-headedness.

2 The following considerations suggest that requesting admission would be appropriate.
   - The patient could benefit from immediate nursing care, and the alternative requests may merely cause delay in admission.
   - Blood tests, ECG, urine and stool tests and X-ray are required for assessment, and are best organized at the hospital. They take time, and it will be more convenient if the patient is admitted for assessment.
   - You can describe the patient's home circumstances, adaptation and degree of dementia to the consultant in the referral letter.

   Having the patient seen at the out-patient department or as a domiciliary might be better if you wish to reduce the risk that she will be admitted to an under-resourced ward and lose the capacity to care for herself.

   The following considerations suggest that requesting a domiciliary visit would be appropriate.
   - Only 50% of patients referred to geriatric out-patients turn up in the ambulance.
   - The patient's level of dementia may deteriorate in a strange environment and cannot be assessed in these circumstances.
   - The domiciliary visit may result in investigations at the day-hospital rather than as an in-patient.
   - Someone from the geriatric team will visit in any case to assess the home situation before the patient is discharged.
   - The patient's untidy home and stained clothes may be due to aggravation of her dementia by the metabolic effects of the current diarrhoea. This might respond quickly to treatment, and a temporary increase in provision of home care could meet her social needs.
   - The geriatrician needs to be able to assess the degree of priority for use of one of their scarce hospital beds.

3 a Whether she is reasonably free of pain, can move all her limbs, and can get water and go to the toilet.
   b Whether she can use medication reliably and take food reliably, whether she is likely to fall again, and whether she should be investigated further.

4 We asked how a doctor should respond when he diagnoses depression in an apathetic, frail, elderly patient but the carer attributes the symptoms to a physical cause and asks for a second opinion. One has to consider whether the carer feels impugned by the doctor's diagnosis, and whether he or she has a true perception of the responsiveness

of this condition to simple treatment. It is obviously worth exploring the carer's views and concerns, and indeed whether the carer is him- or herself depressed, or possibly just does not have the patient's best interests at heart. In the absence of agreement, a prescription for antidepressants is probably futile, but perhaps one can negotiate that the doctor will obtain a second opinion, but would be grateful if the carer could give the benefit of the doubt to the possibility that the patient might respond to an antidepressant. Obtaining a second opinion will involve delay, and there seems little point in denying the patient the possibility of effective treatment in the mean time. A psychogeriatric CPN might be a considerable help in this situation.

5   For many carers a major source of stress is the loss of sleep due to feeling that they have to be alert at night for movement or cries of distress from their invalid relative. The help of a care assistant to sleep next-door to the patient may be much appreciated. For cancer sufferers, Macmillan nurses and the Marie Curie Foundation can sometimes provide this service. For sufferers from stroke or dementia the provision is poor. If the Disabled Living Allowance is insufficient to pay for a night-time care assistant, the Disabled Living Foundation, Age Concern and the Countess Mountbatten Foundation may provide additional financial support. Some families have found a student or other single person willing to take on such duties in return for free lodgings or rent at a discount. However, service does require external supervision.

6   The following is a consensus of views expressed by GPs responding to this question. The fit elderly are well placed to participate in the care of the housebound and invalids. They might have a better understanding than younger carers of the feelings, social history and attitudes of the individual concerned, they might provoke less anxiety than professional carers, and they themselves might benefit from feeling that they have a useful part to play in society. For GPs and practice nurses there would be less need for visits.

What role might GPs have in organizing this? They frequently see both the fit elderly and the invalid elderly, and appear to be well placed to initiate informal links provided that both parties are willing. However, GPs do not have the resources to supervise and maintain such links. Age Concern, Helping Hands and Help the Aged run such schemes in many localities, and doctors might encourage people to use them. Since the Community Care Act 1990 came into operation, social services departments have been required to take responsibility for providing such services, which they increasingly do by contracting them out to voluntary bodies.

7   Exercises for balance:
   • walking heel to toe
   • walking backwards
   • stepping over increasingly large objects
   • standing on one leg
   • dancing.
   Exercises for strengthening:
   • knee flexion/extension and hip abduction/adduction with weights attached to the

ankle (e.g. progressively heavier bags of rice inside a towel knotted around the ankle)

- step-ups to progressively higher platforms
- standing up from progressively lower seats
- knee bends.

8  Postprandial hypotension causing fainting.

9  a  Osteoarthritis, fracture and osteomalacia.

   b  Serum alkaline phosphatase and urinary hydroxyproline excretion. Note that alkaline phosphatase may also be raised in hypovitaminosis D.

   c  Etidronate 5 mg/kg daily for 6 months or 10 mg/kg daily for 3 months, tiludronate 5 mg/kg daily for 3 months.

   d  Repeat measurement of indices of bone formation and resorption at the end of treatment and at intervals thereafter. Remission is considered to continue until indices rise by 25% above the post-treatment level.

10  False – no observable effect on the severity of incontinence was found.

11  a  True.

    b  True.

12  The author suggests vestibular rehabilitation exercises, behavioural or cognitive therapy, a walking stick and, if possible, arranging for a helping companion to encourage her to be more active.

13  True.

14  a  True.

    b  False.

    c  False – it should be taken for 4 weeks to determine how effective it is for the individual patient.

    d  True.

15  Naftidrofuryl.

16  An aortic aneurysm.

# OPHTHALMOLOGY

**1** What simple facilities are needed to ensure a valid measurement of visual acuity using a Snellen chart? (*2 points*)

*BMJ.* **309**: 1408 (short report)

**2** Visual acuity readings on Snellen charts: (*True/False*)

 **a** are subject to greatest imprecision in people with good acuity

 **b** are poor discriminators of a slight reduction in acuity for people with poor acuity

 **c** yield highly reproducible results.

*BMJ.* **310**: 1481–2

**3** Shining a pen torch into the eye from a distance of 15 cm for 2 s is likely to cause pain in the following conditions: (*True/False*)

 **a** conjunctivitis

 **b** keratitis

 **c** anteror uveitis.

*Br J Gen Pract.* **43**: 259 (letter)

**4** Which eye conditions are particularly noticed when the patient is concentrating?

*BMJ.* **304**: 1096–8

**5** Which classes of drugs are useful in the treatment of corneal abrasions? (*2 points*)

*BMJ.* **307**: 1022

**6** Retinal artery occlusion.

 **a** What is appropriate first aid for someone with a central retinal arterial occlusion? (*3 points*)

**b** What two emergency treatments may restore some vision in a patient with a very recent retinal artery occlusion?

*BMJ.* **303**: 1445–6

*BMJ.* **306**: 942

**7** Visual acuity for driving. (*True/False*)

**a** The ability to read a car number plate at 25 yards approximates to 6/18 on the Snellen chart.

**b** The majority of drivers who are told that they should report impaired visual acuity to the DVLC do so.

*BMJ.* **307**: 844–5

**8** Reduced visual acuity in the elderly can only rarely be helped by spectacles. (*True/False*)

*Br J Gen Pract.* **44**: 587–9 (discussion paper)

**9** The following factors may render myopic patients unsuitable for treatment by laser excimer keratectomy: (*True/False*)

**a** age over 30 years

**b** requires perfect vision

**c** user of contact lenses

**d** diabetes

**e** severe myopia ($> -8$ D)

**f** severe astigmatism ($> 2$ D)

**g** occupation involves much night driving

**h** pupils are small in dim light.

*BMJ.* **310**: 979–85

**10** A young adult who uses soft contact lenses has conjunctivitis. How will you advise him to treat the condition and to prevent its recurrence? (*4 points*)

*BMJ.* **308**: 1116–17

**11** Approximately what proportion of people over 40 years of age attending an optometrist are likely to have their intra-ocular pressure checked?

*BMJ.* **302**: 998–1000

**12** What proportion of patients over 65 years of age have had a sight test in the past 3 years?

*BMJ.* **314**: 246 (leading article)

**13** Detecting glaucoma. (*True/False*)

**a** Most patients referred by optometrists after glaucoma screening do not have glaucoma or raised intra-ocular pressure (IOP) when examined by the ophthalmologist.

**b** Glaucoma is commoner in people with severe short sight.

**c** Glaucoma is commoner in Asians.

**d** An IOP of more than 24 mmHg with normal optic disks and visual fields justifies referral to an ophthalmologist.

*BMJ.* **310**: 546–7

**14** Screening for glaucoma with oculokinetic perimetry. (*True/False*)

**a** The prevalence of undetected glaucoma in patients aged 60–80 years is at least 5%.

**b** Normal intra-ocular pressure is found in about 50% of elderly people suffering glaucoma.

**c** About 50% of those who show abnormal results on oculokinetic perimetry are finally considered to have no ocular abnormality.

*Br J Gen Pract.* **43**: 478–9

**15** Which of the following measurements appear useful and practical when screening for glaucoma in general practice? List the procedures in your order of preference.

**a** Intra-ocular pressure.

**b** Oculokinetic perimetry.

**c** Fundoscopy for cup/disc ratio.

*Br J Gen Pract.* **41**: 216–17

**16** It is unsafe to use a mydriatic in a patient with chronic open-angle glaucoma. (*True/False*)

*BMJ.* **310**: 1668

**17** What features of a patient and his or her presentation of a headache might lead you to suspect that acute angle-closure glaucoma is imminent? (*8 or more points*)

*BMJ.* **313**: 413–14 (case reports)

**18** Why may low blood pressure endanger sight? (*1 point*)

*BMJ.* **313**: 1024 (citation)

**19** The diabetic retina. (*True/False*)

a The retinae of newly diagnosed adult diabetics are only rarely abnormal.

b Venous dilatation is a serious sign of impending loss of vision.

c Looped veins indicate a need for intense surveillance.

d Exudates at the macula are an indication for photocoagulation.

e New vessels commonly arise at the margin of the optic disk.

f Vitrectomy may salvage vision after a retinal haemorrhage.

g Aspirin is indicated for advanced retinopathy.

h Retinopathy progresses more slowly during pregnancy.

*BMJ.* **307**: 195–8

**20** How may photocoagulation affect vision? (*2 points*)

*BMJ.* **305**: 1238–9

**21** The following patients may benefit from laser treatment without additional ocular surgery: (*True/False*)

a a 75-year-old with diminishing acuity and no sign of a cataract

b a patient with a detached retina

c a diabetic with lipid deposits near the macula

d a patient with an early cataract

e a patient who has had an intracapsular lens implant and now notes increasingly cloudy vision in the same eye

f a patient with acute glaucoma

g a patient with myopia.

*BMJ.* **304**: 1161–5

**22** Current evidence suggests that oestrogens protect against senile macular degeneration. (*True/False*)

*BMJ.* **310**: 1570–1

**23** Exposure to sunlight is a factor leading to cataract formation. (*True/False*)

*BMJ.* **315**: 136 (citation)

**24** What serum constituents have been found to exist in lower concentration in patients who subsequently developed cataract than in controls? (*2 points*)

*BMJ.* **305**:1392–4

**25** An ophthalmologist complains that his work is inefficient because too many patients are referred to him with raised IOP or as children with squint so mild that it is not clinically relevant. Can you devise criteria for appropriate referral in these two situations?

*BMJ.* **315**: 318 (personal view)

# ANSWERS

1 A spotlight, and a 3 m or 6 m line measure.

2 a True – there are more letters in the lines of smaller print, and the greater proximity of the letters increases the difficulty in reading them.

   b True – 6/60 to 6/24 is a big difference, and many Snellen charts have no line of letters in between.

   c False – 13% of patients record discrepancies of two lines or more at successive readings.

   New Snellen charts have been produced which resolve these problems. Scoring involves recording successful and unsuccessful attempts to read letters throughout the chart, and this is more sensitive to small changes in acuity than merely recording the line at which the patient fails to read the majority of letters.

3 a False.

   b True.

   c True.

4 Dry eyes, blepharitis and macular degeneration.

5 Antibiotic and mydriatic drugs.

6 a Massage the eyes to reduce intra-ocular pressure and cause the embolus to move peripherally. The patient should rebreathe into a bag to build up carbon dioxide levels, and should take acetazolamide.

   b A massive dose of prednisolone and thrombolysis.

7 a False – reading a car number plate at 25 yards approximates to 6/10 on the Snellen chart.

   b False.

8 False.

9 a False – age over 21 years is a precondition for treatment. Patients with presbyopia will need reading glasses after the operation.

   b True.

   c False – contact lens users are preferred as they can use a single contact lens to correct the untreated eye during the interval between correcting the first and second eyes.

   d True.

   e True.

   f True.

   g True.

h False – patients with large pupils may notice haloes around lights after the operation.

10 Treatment – application of neomycin or propamidine will kill all of the most likely pathogens, as well as acanthamoeba, which occasionally causes serious ocular damage. Prevention – sterilize lenses daily in hydrogen peroxide or chlorhexidine. Clean the lens container in boiled water at 70 degrees centigrade. Thiomersal should be avoided both in cleansing solutions and in treatment, as it occasionally causes hypersensitivity.

11 About 50%.

12 An average figure is 37%, although the proportion is much lower in the unskilled than in professional people.

13 a False – 55% do.

   b True – and in people with long sight.

   c False – more commoner in Afro-Caribbeans.

   d False – an IOP of 26 mmHg in the absence of other features of glaucoma justifies referral.

14 a True.

   b True.

   c True.

15 • Intra-ocular pressure – widely regarded as a poor predictor of retinal damage with considerable variation on successive observations.

   • Perimetry – easily administered with good specificity and able to identify those with retinal damage (i.e. those who can benefit from treatment). However, the method is not yet well validated.

   • Cup/disc ratio – the findings of inexperienced observers may be unreliable.

16 False – narrow-angle glaucoma which poses a danger is an acute condition that requires urgent surgical treatment. Individuals with a known history of glaucoma have open-angle glaucoma.

17 Long-sighted patient, female patient, recent introduction of an anticholinergic drug, headache associated with blurring of vision or haloes around lights, headache worse in semi-darkness, unilateral or frontal headache followed by painful red eye, fixed semi-dilated pupil, and reduced acuity.

18 If the blood pressure dips below the intra-ocular pressure, the blood supply to the optic nerve may be endangered, causing glaucomatous damage.

19 a False.

   b False.

   c True.

   d True.

   e True.

   f True.

**g** False.

**h** True.

20 It may cause impaired peripheral vision and dark adaptation.

21 **a** True.

**b** False.

**c** True.

**d** False.

**e** True.

**f** True.

**g** True.

22 True – early menopause increases the risk and HRT has been found to reduce it.

23 True.

24 Alpha-tocopherol and beta-carotene.

25 The ophthalmologist writing in the *British Medical Journal* complained that excessive time is used at his clinics in checking for glaucoma in patients with slightly raised intra-ocular pressures and in checking for squint in children with only very mild forms of the disorder.

Doctors addressing this question suggested that there should be greater provision of technical workers at the eye clinic, in order to avoid medical time being used for routine predictable measurements. Perhaps high-street optometrists could be better trained to rescreen patients suspected of having glaucoma with optokinetic perimetry and fundoscopy, as well as repeat IOP measurements.

Doctors also suggested that squints should only be referred if the child is over 2 years of age and has a continuous squint, or if at any age there is any evidence of reduced acuity in one eye.

# ORTHOPAEDICS

**1** What can a GP do to minimize the risk of infection in a prosthetic hip joint?

*BMJ.* **309**: 506–7

**2** Bony problems.

**a** A 13-year-old girl notes pain under her forefoot on weight-bearing, but there is no history of trauma or sudden stress. There is local tenderness, swelling and pain on extending the middle toes. What is the likely diagnosis and what initial treatment is appropriate?

**b** A patient reports pain in the hindfoot, and on examination there is rigidity of movement at the subtalar joint. What condition may be revealed by X-ray or CT examination?

**c** A teenage cricket bowler complains of low back pain. Why is it important to X-ray his spine?

*BMJ.* **308**: 1556–9

*BMJ.* **309**: 79

**3** What type of fall may produce a fractured scaphoid?

*BMJ.* **310**: 239–43 (review)

**4** Immobilization in plaster of Paris is the best treatment for a scaphoid fracture. (*True/False*)

*BMJ.* **315**: 68 (citation)

**5** What type of patient might benefit from acetabular redirection?

*BMJ.* **315**: 265–6 (leading article)

**6** What information should patients who have orthopaedic implants or prostheses carry around with them in case they require further surgery at the same site in an emergency?

*BMJ.* **315**: 1377 (letter)

**7**    Most hip arthroplasties are still functional after 25 years. (*True/False*)

*BMJ.* **316**: 320 (citation)

**8**    What incidence of deep vein thrombosis after arthroscopic surgery of the knee has been quoted?

*BMJ.* **316**: 562 (citation)

**9**    What is the probability of a patient with osteoarthritis of the knee that is unresponsive to medication deriving benefit from arthroscopy?

*BMJ.* **304**: 94

# ANSWERS

1 Treat oral sepsis and advise on dentistry before the operation. Encourage the patient to maintain good oral hygiene thereafter.

2   a Freiberg's disease. The appropriate initial treatment would be rest and a metatarsal pad bar. X-ray to exclude loose bodies, and if the latter are present, consider referral to a podiatric surgeon for removal of loose fragments.

    b Calcaneonavicular bar or talonavicular bar.

    c Fracture of the pars-interarticularis of the lower lumbar vertebra may be the cause. It heals best with immobilization in a plastic jacket.

3 A fall on an outstretched arm with the wrist extended.

4 False – a minimally invasive percutaneous method of screw fixation using a guide wire and an image intensifier gets the patient back to work more quickly.

5 A patient with acetabular dysplasia, usually a female presenting with early onset of pain in the hip on weight-bearing, usually unrestricted in range of movement, and with a shallow maldirected acetabulum on X-ray.

6 The patient's hospital number, the date, site and type of implant, relevant comments, and the manufacturer's name.

7 True – 81% of the femoral components and 68% of the acetabular components in this report had survived for 25 years.

8 33 of 184 patients developed deep vein thrombosis after arthroscopy, and it was symptomatic in 20 of these patients.

9 60–80%.

# PAIN

## Diagnosis

**1** Migraine headaches are characteristically aggravated by movement. (*True/False*)

*BMJ.* **312**: 1279–83 (review)

**2** What is the best laboratory index of the activity of giant-cell arteritis to use in general practice?

*BMJ.* **305**: 68–9

**3** What information would help to determine whether a pain in the arm in an individual patient is related to his or her occupation by association or by causation?

*BMJ.* **304**: 309–11

**4** What findings on history and physical examination support a diagnosis of pain due to dysfunction of the musculoskeletal system rather than structural abnormality?

*Br J Gen Pract.* **47**: 653–5 (discussion paper)

## Management

**1** How can you reduce the pain of a local anaesthetic injection?

*BMJ.* **305**: 617–18

**2** What dosage regime of prednisolone is appropriate for most patients with giant cell arteritis?

*BMJ.* **305**: 68–9

**3** What quicker-acting alternative to EMLA cream is available for topical anaesthesia before cannulation?

*BMJ.* **314**: 201–3 (review)

**4** What first-aid treatment and what curative treatment would you suggest for a patient who suffers a severe headache, relieved by lying down, 48 h after an epidural anaesthetic? (*2 points*)

*BMJ.* **306**: 874–5

**5** List four or more treatments worthy of consideration for a patient with pain in the face, when investigations have failed to reveal an organic cause.

*BMJ.* **304**: 329–30

**6** The writer of this letter suggests that many patients with chronic pain of benign origin respond to cognitive behavioural treatment. With limited time at your disposal, what key concepts would you seek to communicate at a first consultation on this topic? (*4 points*)

*BMJ.* **306**: 1687–8

**7** What warning on use do you give to patients when prescribing minor analgesics for a chronic intermittent tension headache? (*2 or more points*)

*BMJ.* **310**: 479–80

**8** Amitriptyline for pain.
  **a** For which painful conditions is there good evidence that amitriptyline is an effective treatment?
  **b** What is the median preferred dose for analgesic effect?
  **c** How soon is the onset of action?

*BMJ.* **314**: 763–4 (leading article)

**9** Pain management. (*True/False*)
  **a** Ibuprofen is more effective than paracetamol.
  **b** Pethidine is better than other opioids for colicky pain.
  **c** Opioids may cause urinary retention.

*BMJ.* **314**: 1531–5 (review article)

**10** In a Health Technology Board review of control of chronic pain:

  **a** what topical treatment has been found to be likely to help pain of diabetic neuropathy?

  **b** what injected treatment is likely to be helpful for lumbago/sciatica?

  **c** what psychological treatment has been found helpful for many mental health problems associated with chronic pain?

  *BMJ.* **315**: 274 (news item)

**11** If escalating doses of morphine and co-analgesics are not controlling neuropathic cancer pain, or are causing intolerable side-effects, what alternatives exist that are specific for the N-methyl D-aspartate receptor? (*2 points*)

  *BMJ.* **316**: 81 (letter)

**12** What advice on self-management might help a tense person with temporo-mandibular joint pain?

  *BMJ.* **316**: 190–3 (review)

**13** What is a suitable starting dose of morphine to relieve pain from a fracture in a frail elderly person, in the experience of this consultant physician?

  *BMJ.* **316**: 281 (letter)

# ANSWERS

## Diagnosis

1 True.

2 C-reactive protein may be better than the conventional ESR as it is not affected by anaemia and is more stable if there is a delay between sampling and measurement.

3 Complaints of stiffness in the hand and forearm after prolonged writing, typing or use of hand-tools are common. GPs may be asked to advise these patients on whether the pains are work related and whether it is wise to change job, retire early or even report or sue the employer. As the article mentions, there have been no controlled studies of microscopic or neurophysiological changes in these cases. However, since this article was published there have been reports of thermograms of the hands revealing changes in sufferers among patients with repetitive strain syndrome. In the absence of such evidence we are left observing whether the patients' symptoms and signs correspond to a recognized anatomical pattern or recognized syndrome and assessing whether boredom or alienation from the employment are contributing to the complaint.

   A pain diary with an account of activities that preceded the pain might be useful in individual cases. If similar symptoms and temporal associations with similar work are found in pain diaries from several sufferers recording independently, and if the patients appear otherwise to enjoy good physical and mental health, an occupational association becomes more likely.

   It may be instructive to obtain a report from the employer or the occupational health adviser.

4 History – the patient may complain of pain experienced after an awkward movement, overuse, or on waking. Pain is often referred distally, aggravated by particular postures and activities, and relieved by rest and lying down. Other features are unduly prolonged pain or hypersensitivity after application of painful stimuli (hyperaesthesia), and pain in response to stimuli that are not normally painful (allodynia).
Examination – bilateral asymmetry, reduced range of joint movement, localized tenderness, reduced resistance to tracking a finger over the affected area due to increased sweating, oedema under the skin and thickening due to spasm of muscle may be palpable.

# Management

1   Warm the syringe to 37 degrees centigrade.

2   If vision is threatened start with 500 mg of intravenous methylprednisolone and 80 mg prednisolone daily thereafter. In the absence of a threat to vision, start with 20 mg prednisolone daily and taper this slowly to 10 mg/day. Thereafter the dose should be reduced by 1 mg/day at monthly intervals unless symptoms reappear. However, many patients require a low maintenance dose for years. The need for steroid may be reduced by taking a dose of a non-steroidal drug or codeine to cover the early hours of the morning.

3   4% amethocaine gel (Ametop 1.5 g tubes), also used for analgesia before cryotherapy.

4   First aid – an abdominal binder.
    Curative – epidural injection of 10–20 mL of autologous blood.

5   Antidepressants, vitamin $B_1$ (for burning pain in the mouth), low-dose neuroleptics, and psychological treatments such as relaxation, behaviour therapy, cognitive therapy or biofeedback.

6   Patients with a chronic pain of benign origin may enjoy a better quality of life if they develop appropriate attitudes to their problem and limit their consumption of sedative analgesics. Doctors responding to this question suggested advising such patients as follows.

   • Give reassurance that the doctor is familiar with the problem, realizes that the pain is real, and is sympathetic.

   • Emphasize that the pain is due to a benign cause, it will not cause death or severe disability, and it may improve with time.

   • Suggest that the patient should not allow the pain to control his or her life, and should try to crowd it out with other pleasures and pursuits.

   • Suggest avoiding self-pity. People can get on with their lives despite pain.

   • Use relaxation and distraction techniques when the pain comes on.

   • Be open about the pain to people around you. Help them to realize that it imposes some disability but that this is tolerable.

   • Do not use tablets unless they really help. However, the doctor will not cut off the supply if the patient is finding them useful.

   • Try a TENS machine or an ultrasound or vibrating massager. Doctors can not always predict whether these will help, but they are effective for some people.

7   The author's suggestion is that, to avoid an analgesic-associated headache, analgesic should not be used for more than 15 days per month. In the case of migraine headaches treated with ergotamine or sumatriptan, these should not be used for more than 10 days per month.

**8 a** Established post-herpetic neuralgia (1 in 2.3 cases achieved 50% pain relief in 3–6 weeks), diabetic neuropathy (1 in 3 cases achieved 50% pain relief), atypical facial pain (1 in 2.8 cases achieved 50% pain relief), and pain after stroke (1 in 1.7 cases).

   **b** Median preferred dose is 75 mg amitriptyline.

   **c** Onset of action occurs in 1–7 days.

   **d** Benefits have also been reported with regard to fibromyalgia, irritable bowel syndrome and temporomandibular joint pain.

**9 a** True.

   **b** False.

   **c** True.

**10 a** Capsaicin.

   **b** Lumbar epidural with corticosteroid.

   **c** Cognitive behavioural therapy.

**11** Accumulation of morphine-3–glucuronide may cause stimulatory side-effects. Methadone and ketamine are specific for the N-methyl D-aspartate receptor, and methadone is also an agonist at the $\mu$-receptor.

**12** Cultivate relaxation of the jaw muscles. Eat soft foods. Massage may help. Use a gumshield if prone to tooth-grinding during sleep. Use analgesics or minor tranquillizers on a regular basis for a finite period.

**13** 1–2 mg every 4 h, together with a laxative. The final dose varies considerably, but the physician reports no difficulty in withdrawing morphine when symptoms abate.

# RHEUMATOLOGY

## Aetiology

**1** What type of alcoholic drink is most likely to provoke gout?

*BMJ.* **309**: 680

**2** Which vaccines may cause a transient polyarthritis? (*3 points*)

*BMJ.* **310**: 1128–32

**3** Why may middle-aged patients with backache due to osteoarthritis be less likely to have osteoporosis than others?

*BMJ.* **302**: 602

**4** What diseases may underlie Raynaud's phenomenon in an elderly person? (*3 points*)

*BMJ.* **310**: 239–43 (review)

**5** What organism has been identified in the joints of people with rheumatoid disease and inflammatory joint disease of unknown origin?

*BMJ.* **310**: 239–43 (review)

*BMJ.* **313**: 1024 (citation)

**6** What is Costen's syndrome – and to what disease processes is it attributable?

*BMJ.* **315**: 1632 (citation)

**7** What demographic group is prone to inflammation at the pubic insertion of the inguinal ligament?

*BMJ.* **309**: 1592 (citation)

**8** What other part of the body is subject to contracture with a histological similarity to Dupuytren's contracture?

*BMJ* **314**: 1562 (citation)

**9** What physiological response to 5 min of typing has been shown in almost all patients with repetitive strain syndrome, but much less commonly in controls?

*BMJ.* **314**: 118 (research report)

# Diagnosis

**1** How might a GP rate the severity of a frozen shoulder? List three or more useful observations which the doctor could obtain from the patient or could make him- or herself.

*BMJ.* **302**: 1498–51

*BMJ.* **303**: 123

**2** In a patient with a painful shoulder not related to any injury, and with no neck stiffness, what is the significance of the following clinical features?

**a** Pain is localized to the upper arm and is felt when the patient lies on the affected side. There is a painful arc on passive and active abduction, and external rotation is limited.

**b** There is a painful arc on active abduction but not on passive abduction.

**c** Pain is localized to the top of the shoulder and the suprascapular area, and is aggravated by passive horizontal adduction and passive extension of the abducted arm.

*BMJ.* **310**: 183–6 (review)

**3** What should one check for when examining and investigating a patient with Raynaud's phenomenon? (*4 points*)

*BMJ.* **310**: 795–8

**4** What investigation will reveal the best evidence of prognosis in a patient with acute systemic vasculitis?

*BMJ.* **310**: 1128–32

**5** Can you provide a diagnosis and treatment for the following patients with painful feet?

**a** There is gradual onset of burning pain while walking, in the third and fourth toes, in a middle-aged woman. Pressure at the base of the painful cleft produces pain and a click.

**b** A 13-year-old boy who plays a lot of football has pain at the base of one toe when he steps off with that foot, and he limps as a result. The toe looks swollen, and pulling the toe brings on the pain.

**c** A man who has recently done a lot of hill-walking notes pain under his heel that is made worse by compression. The part looks swollen.

*BMJ.* **310**: 860–4

**6** Rheumatoid arthritis.

**a** What conditions other than rheumatoid arthritis may be associated with a positive rheumatoid factor? (*6 points*)

**b** Which nerves are particularly subject to nerve entrapment in rheumatoid arthritis? (*4 points*)

*BMJ.* **310**: 587–90, 637–40, 652–5, 1139

**7** Fibromyalgia. (*True/False*)

**a** Pain may be particularly noted on withdrawal of pressure.

**b** Pain is always well localized.

**c** Poor sleep is characteristic.

*BMJ.* **310**: 386–9

**8** Gout. (*True/False*)

**a** In a patient with a painful foot a high uric acid level is sufficient justification for a diagnosis of gout.

**b** Uric acid deposition is a common cause of renal failure, and thiazide diuretics are the initial treatment of choice.

*BMJ.* **310**: 521–4

**9** Which painful conditions of the knee may be diagnosed from an MRI scan? (*8 points*)

*BMJ.* **311**: 1614 (research report)

**10** A patient develops severe polyarthralgia 2 weeks after an attack of enteritis.

**a** What blood investigation is of most prognostic value?

**b** What investigations may yield a result suggesting a specific treatment? (*2 points*)

*BMJ.* **308**: 671–2

**11** Polyarthralgia of recent onset. (*True/False*)

**a** Investigations for rheumatoid arthritis should be delayed for 6 weeks.

**b** Rheumatoid arthritis is extremely unlikely if distal interphalangeal joints are involved.

*Br J Gen Pract.* **47**: 469 (review of review)

**12** Paget's disease.

**a** What other diseases does the pain produced mimic? (*2 points*)

**b** What routine biochemical tests are useful if screening for the condition? (*2 points*)

*BMJ.* **312**: 491–4 (review)

**13** Septic arthritis in a patient with osteoarthritis.

**a** What conditions predispose to this complication?

**b** What symptom results?

**c** What findings confirm the diagnosis?

*BMJ.* **313**: 40–1 (case reports)

**14** 'Doctor, my shoulders ache for an hour or two in the mornings and now I'm getting a throbbing pain at the side of my head.'

**a** What other clinical features of giant cell arteritis might you probe for as you take a more detailed history from this old lady? *(10 or more points)*

**b** What abnormalities may be seen in the fundus if arteries supplying the fundus are involved? (*2 points*)

*BMJ.* **314**: 1329–32 (review)

**15** Giant cell arteritis. (*True/False*)

**a** It commonly affects the occipital artery.

**b** The ESR is always raised.

**c** Temporal artery biopsy may be positive in the absence of symptoms.

**d** Histological inflammation of the temporal artery takes several weeks to respond to steroids.

*BMJ.* **310**: 1057–9

# Management

**1** What percentage of patients in general practice with shoulder pain, most of whom are treated with steroid injections, would you expect to be completely relieved of the problem at 6 months and at 18 months?

*BMJ.* **313**: 601 (study report)

**2** Physiotherapy for soft-tissue shoulder disorders is well supported by trial evidence of efficacy. (*True/False*)

*BMJ.* **315**: 25–9 (systematic review)

**3** What else apart from kidney stones may lithotriptors be useful for?

*BMJ.* **316**: 154 (citation)

**4** What device in the home might help a sufferer from rotator cuff injury to mobilize the shoulder? (*1 point*)

*BMJ.* **307**: 899–900

**5** Intra-articular injections of the glenohumeral joint. (*True/False*)

**a** They only provide relief if the fluid is delivered into the joint.

**b** If no synovial fluid can be withdrawn into the syringe the injection is almost certain to be extra-articular.

*BMJ.* **307**: 1329–30

**6** After a steroid injection for tennis elbow:

**a** what percentage of patients experience temporary worsening of the pain?

**b** what percentage of patients experience skin atrophy?

**c** how long does relief from pain typically last?

*Br J Gen Pract.* **46**: 209–16 (meta-analysis)

**7** How should the needle be directed when injecting steroid for carpal tunnel syndrome? (*3 points*)

*BMJ.* **310**: 239–43 (review)

**8** Oestrogen treatment is likely to exacerbate carpal tunnel syndrome. (*True/False*)

*BMJ.* **303**: 1514

**9** Supplements of what vitamin have been reported to help people with carpal tunnel syndrome?

*BMJ.* **310**: 1534

**10** In what situations are intra-articular steroid injections justified for a patient with an inflamed knee? (*3 points*)

*BMJ.* **310**: 457–61

**11** Most patients with osteoarthritis of the knee notice a benefit when a tape is applied to pull the patella medially. How quickly does the effect develop?

*BMJ.* **308**: 753–5

**12** What is the probability that a patient with osteoarthritis of the knee that is unresponsive to medication will derive benefit from arthroscopy?

*BMJ.* **304**: 94

**13** Arthroscopy may be a suitable investigation and treatment for patients with the following conditions: (*True/False*)

**a** shoulder impingement syndrome

**b** a loose body in the elbow

**c** a 45-year-old man with degenerative disease of the hip

**d** fusion of a chronically painful ankle

**e** rheumatoid disease of the metacarpophalangeal joints.

*BMJ.* **308**: 51–3

**14** The following patients with severe knee pain may suitably be referred for total knee replacement: (*True/False*)

**a** a 66-year-old man with osteoarthritis of the knee and gross enlargement and derangement of the knee on X-ray, who has a sedentary lifestyle and only notices knee pain when he is shopping

**b** a 40-year-old housewife with nocturnal and early morning pain due to rheumatoid disease of the knee

**c** a 55-year-old dustman with osteoarthritis of the knee who frequently needs time off work because of the pain.

*BMJ.* **303**: 262

**15** Non-steroidal anti-inflammatory drugs have been found to delay fracture healing in animal studies. (*True/False*)

*BMJ.* **306**: 1493

**16** Non-steroidal anti-inflammatory drugs are the treatment of choice for soft-tissue injuries. (*True/False*)

*BMJ.* **31**: 206

**17** Tendonitis.

**a** Non-steroidal drugs and a local steroid injection are not relieving an acute crepitating tendonitis. What other medical treatment is effective?

**b** Medical treatment and physiotherapy are not relieving severe shoulder tendonitis. What operation may relieve nocturnal pain?

*BMJ.* **313**: 419–22 (review)

**18** What advice to patients seems likely to reduce the incidence of NSAID-associated gastro-intestinal bleeds?

*BMJ.* **316**: 492 (editorial)

**19** Rheumatology.

**a** Where are cyclo-oxygenases 1 and 2 found?

**b** By how much do long-acting anti-inflammatories reduce long-term dis-ability in rheumatoid arthritis?

*BMJ.* **316**: 1810–12 (review)

**20** Rheumatoid arthritis.

**a** What proportion of patients treated with sulphasalazine, penicillamine or injectable gold achieve good long-term control and improved function?

**b** If prednisolone is used as treatment, what appears to be the minimal effective dose?

**c** When intra-articular steroids are used, what determines whether a depot preparation or a short-acting injection of hydrocortisone or prednisolone should be used? (*3 points*)

**d** When methotrexate is used, what drug interaction will restrict the choice of antibacterial agent that can be used for incidental infections? (*1 point*)

*BMJ.* **310**: 587–90, 637–40, 652–5, 1139

**21** What antibiotic has been shown to be of clinical benefit for patients with rheumatoid arthritis?

*BMJ.* **310**: 610

**22** What side-effects may be encountered and what monitoring is required during therapy with the following drugs for rheumatoid arthritis?

**a** Hydroxychloroquine.

**b** Sulphasalazine.

*BMJ.* **307**: 425–8

*BMJ.* **316**: 716–17 (leading article)

**23** Disease-modifying drugs in rheumatoid arthritis. (*True/False*)

**a** Early introduction is associated with improved clinical measures and lower erythrocyte sedimentation rates.

**b** Early introduction is associated wth a better radiological outcome after 5 years.

*BMJ.* **314**: 766–17 (leading article)

**24** Fibromyalgia. (*True/False*)

**a** A non-steroidal anti-inflammatory drug is likely to be effective.

**b** Patients should be encouraged to live within the limits set by their pain.

**c** Most patients will recover within 5 years.

*BMJ.* **310**: 386–9

**25** Gout. (*True/False*)

**a** A high uric acid level is enough to justify lifelong treatment with allo-purinol.

**b** A high dose of prednisolone administered by injection is effective for acute gout.

**c** An NSAID is required only for the first week or two when allopurinol is introduced.

**d** Allopurinol may prevent renal stones other than uric acid stones.

*BMJ.* **310**: 521–4

**26** What is an appropriate dose of allopurinol for someone with a creatinine clearance rate of 10 mL/min?

*BMJ.* **312**: 173–4 (case report and discussion)

**27** Paget's disease.

**a** For how long should oral biphosphonate treatment be continued? (*2 points*)

**b** What monitoring is useful thereafter? (*2 points*)

*BMJ.* **312**: 491–4 (review)

# ANSWERS

## Aetiology

1 Beer – as it may have a high content of guanosine.

2 Influenza, rubella and tetanus toxoid.

3 Exercise may delay osteoporosis while exacerbating osteoarthritis.

4 Rheumatoid arthritis, systemic lupus erythematosus and scleroderma.

5 *Mycoplasma.*

6 Dysfunction of the temporomandibular joint, earache, tinnitus and loss of hearing, attributable variously to osteoarthritis, myofascial pain and psychological stress and anxiety.

7 Athletic young men.

8 Rotator cuff and coracohumeral ligament of the shoulder – frozen shoulder.

9 Cooling of the skin over the proximal phalanges shown on thermography.

## Diagnosis

1 • Use of analgesics.
  • Pain severity at rest on a point scale.
  • Pain on resisted movement.
  • Range of active and passive movement.

2 a Glenohumeral injury or inflammation or adhesive capsulitis – consider a hydrocortisone injection into the subacromial bursa if it does not respond to rest and anti-inflammatories.

  b Rotator cuff tendinitis – consider a hydrocortisone injection into the subacromial bursa.

  c Probable inflammation at the acromioclavicular joint – consider a hydrocortisone injection into this joint if it does not respond to anti-inflammatories.

3 • Neck tenderness suggestive of a cervical rib.
  • Blood pressure in both arms.
  • Peripheral pulses.
  • Antinuclear antibodies.

4  Urinalysis for proteinuria and haematuria.

5  a  Morton's metatarsalgia due to inflammation of the interdigital nerve and plantar digital artery. Suitable footwear and an arch support may help, as may injection of local anaesthetic and steroid around the nerve.

   b  Freiberg's disease due to aseptic infarction and necrosis of the epiphysis at the MTP joint. Rest and immobilization are needed, and some patients benefit from corrective surgery.

   c  Plantar calcaneal bursitis. Rest, anti-inflammatory drugs and medial arch supports are likely to help, as may ultrasound treatment or short-wave diathermy.

6  a  Other connective tissue diseases, viral infections, leprosy, leishmaniasis, subacute bacterial endocarditis, tuberculosis, liver disease, sarcoidosis and mixed essential cryoglobulinaemia.

   b  Median, ulnar, lateral popliteal and tarsal nerves.

7  a  True.

   b  False.

   c  True.

8  a  False – high uric acid levels are quite common in the absence of gout. A diagnosis of gout would require a characteristic X-ray and preferably also the finding of uric acid crystals in a specimen of synovial fluid.

   b  False – uric acid stones are an unlikely cause of renal failure. Confusion arises because impaired renal excretion of uric acid raises plasma levels and may cause gout.

9  Menisceal and ligamentous tears, degenerate menisci, loose bodies, Baker's cyst, osteoarthritis, effusion, chondromalacia patellae, partial ligamentous tears, bursitis and osteochondritis dissecans.

10  a  Some 60–90% of patients with reactive arthritis after an enteric or venereal infection are positive for HLA-B27. Usually their arthritis is asymmetric and monoarticular with painful tendon insertions as well as joints. A minority of them also develop mucocutaneous inflammation, ocular symptoms, urethritis and carditis. The prognosis is worse if the patient is HLA-B27 positive. Symptoms may begin to improve gradually after a few months, but 15–30% of cases develop prolonged arthritis.

    b  High or rising titres of antibodies to *Yersinia* in a patient with postenteric arthritis suggest that 3 months of treatment with lymecycline may be of benefit. Treating any chlamydial infection of the genitalia may also reduce the duration of arthritis.

11  a  True – viral aetiology is more likely and the symptom is usually transient.

    b  True.

12  a  Osteoarthritis, fracture, osteomalacia.

    b  Serum alkaline phosphatase, urinary hydroxyproline excretion. Note that alkaline phosphatase may also be raised in hypovitaminosis D.

13 a Infection, particularly in internal organs.

   b Increasing pain.

   c ESR and CRP, X-ray, joint aspiration and culture.

14 a • Systemic symptoms – night sweats, fatigue, loss of appetite, depression.
  - Pain in the neck and buttocks as well as the shoulders.
  - Tender points noted when brushing the hair, or elsewhere in the side of the head.
  - Jaw or facial pain on chewing.
  - Painless visual loss noted when the patient wakes up.
  - Stroke, myocardial infarction.

   b Splinter haemorrhages and disc oedema.

15 a True.

   b False.

   c True.

   d False – inflammation is reduced within a few days, so biopsy has to be performed quickly after starting steroid treatment for a conclusive diagnosis.

# Management

1 From the results of this study, 21% at 6 months and 58% at 18 months.

2 False.

3 Calcific tendinitis of the shoulder.

4 A sling suspended at shoulder level which bears the weight of the arm as the patient rotates the shoulder.

5 a False – in this study 52% of injections shown by X-ray contrast medium to be directed into the shoulder joint provided relief, but so did 35% of injections shown to be extra-articular.

   b False – in this study it was possible to withdraw synovial fluid prior to only 68% of the injections which were shown by X-ray contrast medium to be intra-articular.

6 a 10–50%.

   b 10–30%.

   c Typically 6–12 weeks.

7 The needle should be inserted at the ulnar side of the tendon of palmaris longus, at the proximal palmar crease and directed forwards at an angle of 45 degrees.

8 False – on the contrary, HRT appears to improve it.

9 Pyridoxine – vitamin $B_6$. Doses of 50–200 mg/day as pyridoxal phosphate relieve the symptoms and have been associated with symptomatic improvement and improved median nerve conduction. Treatment may be required for 3 months, giving cure rates of 85%.

10 The author suggests acute flare-ups of osteoarthritis, patients with osteoarthritis unfit for surgery, and crystal deposition.

11 Within 2 days.

12 60–80% in this study.

13 a True.
  b True.
  c True.
  d True.
  e False.

14 a False – X-ray findings are a poor predictor of benefit.
  b True.
  c True.

15 True.

16 False – no effect on pain or swelling was found when NSAIDs were used as an adjuvant to physiotherapy for hamstring injuries.

17 a Heparin 15 000 units IV daily for 3–4 days.
  b Excision of the lateral part of the acromion.

18 NSAIDs cause irritation of the stomach lining, and they are for symptom relief only, so there is no need to take them if you are free of symptoms. If you note discomfort in the stomach while taking them, stop them and let the doctor know.

19 a Cyclo-oxygenase 1 is found in the gastrointestinal mucosa and kidney. Cyclo-oxygenase 2 is found in inflamed tissue, brain and colon cancers.
  b 30%.

20 a One-third.
  b 5–7.5 mg (at lower doses inadequate control of the disease may reduce mobility and exacerbate osteoporosis).
  c Depot preparations are appropriate for deep injections into major joints, but carry a risk of causing atrophy of skin or subcutaneous tissues when injected into superficial joints or tendon sheaths. In these situations hydrocortisone or pre-dnisolone may be preferable although more painful.
  d Methotrexate is an antifolate drug, so sulphonamides and trimethoprim are likely to be ineffective.

21 Minocycline.

22 a Retinal toxicity – visual acuity, fundoscopy and a central visual field test at the start

of treatment. Issue the patient with an Amsler chart to use on a monthly basis, and ask them to report any abnormality. If treatment is continued for more than 6 years, ophthalmic examination every 6 months may be needed.

b Nausea, skin rash, mouth ulcers, leucopenia, agranulocytosis, reduced sperm count – FBC every 2 weeks for 3 months, then monthly for 3 months, and every 6 weeks thereafter. LFTs every 6 weeks.

23 a True.

b True – but only in those patients for whom NSAIDs did not provide effective relief.

24 a False.

b False.

c False.

25 a False – some patients continue to have high uric acid levels for years without suffering either gout or renal problems. Two-thirds of the purine load comes from the diet so a low-purine diet combined with avoidance of low-dose aspirin and alcohol is recommended.

b True.

c False.

d True.

26 100 mg every 2 days. Allopurinol is all renally excreted, and doses should be reduced proportionally with creatinine clearance if the kidneys are failing.

27 a Etidronate 5 mg/kg daily for 6 months, or 10 mg/kg daily for 3 months, tiludronate 5 mg/kg daily for 3 months.

b Repeat measurement of indices of bone formation and resorption at the end of treatment and at intervals thereafter. Remission is considered to continue until indices have risen by 25% above the post-treatment level.

# SEXUAL AND GENITOURINARY MEDICINE

## Sexual medicine

**1** Parenting is an important influence on a child's sexual orientation. (*True/ False*)

*BMJ.* **303**: 295–6

**2** What topics could usefully be presented in a course or discussion of sex education with teenagers?

*BMJ.* **303**: 992

**3** What techniques seem to be most effective for conveying information on sexual health to teenagers? (*4 points*)

*BMJ.* **311**:1226 (letter)

**4** What proportion of white middle-class women who had recently given birth reported dyspareunia in this survey?

*Br J Gen Pract.* **46**: 47–8

**5** A diabetic aged 45 years complains of erectile impotence. What matters might you discuss and what treatments might you suggest?

*BMJ.* **307**: 738–9

**6** Drugs and the male orgasm.
  **a** What drug may enhance the sensation of orgasm?
  **b** What effect may alpha-blocking drugs used for prostatic obstruction have on sexual function?
  **c** What effect may SSRIs have on male sexual function?

*BMJ.* **314**: 319–20 (leading article)

**7** | Male erectile dysfunction. (*True/False*)

   **a** It reliably improves with restoration of normal testosterone levels.

   **b** It may be improved in patients with deficient testosterone by correction of concomitant hypoprolactinaemia.

   **c** Antihypertensives that are alpha-blockers adversely affect the problem.

   *BMJ.* **316**: 678–81 (review)

**8** | Male erectile dysfunction.

   **a** List the commonly used drugs that may cause the problem.

   **b** What simple questions may rule out organic causes for the problem?

   **c** What physical observations are most important when assessing the problem?

   **d** How does sildenafil work?

   **e** What type of patient is most likely to find vacuum devices acceptable?

   *BMJ.* **316**: 678–81 (review)

**9** | Sildenafil.

   **a** When should it be taken for maximal effect on potency?

   **b** What are its commonest side-effects? (*5 points*)

   *BMJ.* **316**: 1112 (news item)

**10** | What alternative to injection appears to be effective as a delivery system for alprostadil in the treatment of erectile dysfunction?

   *BMJ.* **314**: 238 (citation)

**11** | The following are likely causes of failure of ejaculation. (*True/False*)

   **a** Transurethral resection of the prostate.

   **b** Tricyclic antidepressants.

   **c** Alpha-adrenergic-blockers.

   *BMJ.* **312**: 695–8 (review)

**12** | Subfertility.

   **a** For how long should a man refrain from sexual activity before providing a specimen for semen analysis?

   **b** In a subfertile woman with a low level of progesterone 5 days before her period, what therapeutic inferences would you draw from the following associated features:

    i high levels of follicle-stimulating hormone (FSH) and luteinizing hormone (LH)

    ii high levels of LH but normal FSH together with high androgen levels

    iii borderline high prolactin?

**c** What treatment can be offered to a woman with endometriosis leading to tubal blockage?

**d** What preparations should be made to maximize the success rate of intra-uterine insemination?

**e** For what cause of infertility is *in vitro* fertilization preferable to intra-uterine insemination?

**f** What is the success rate of *in vitro* fertilization?

**g** What is the success rate of intracytoplasmic sperm injection?

*Br J Gen Pract.* **97**: 111–16 (review)

---

**13**    **a** How may a subfertile man feel about this problem?

       **b** How might a GP help him to maintain his morale?

*BMJ.* **316**: 1405–6 (leading article)

---

**14**    Male subfertility.

       **a** What is the most common abnormality found on examination or investigation in men with low sperm counts?

       **b** How effective is surgical treatment for this condition in restoring fertility?

       **c** What advice should be given to a man with a low sperm count to maximize his fertility?

*BMJ.* **306**: 1438–41 (review)

# Genitourinary medicine

**1**    Vaginal candidiasis.

       **a** At what stage of the menstrual cycle are symptoms likely to be worst?

       **b** What is the differential diagnosis of a vaginal itch with no discharge?

       **c** Under what circumstances should a vaginal swab be taken from a woman who presents with symptoms of thrush?

       **d** Which particular symptoms may justify initial use of an oral treatment?

**e** In a woman with recurrent candidiasis, what is the significance of culturing *Candida glabrata* from a vaginal swab?

*BMJ.* **310**: 1241–4

**2** Genital chlamydial infection.

**a** What proportion of pelvic inflammatory disease does this account for?

**b** What benefit has been demonstrated from screening for the condition in young women using conventional assay techniques?

**c** What new assay technique has improved the sensitivity of testing, and what types of samples may it be used on?

**d** What advantage does azithromycin treatment have over earlier antibiotics which justifies its higher cost?

*BMJ.* **313**:1160 (editorial)

**3** What prevalence of chlamydial infection would you expect in endocervical swabs from women under 35 years of age with the following characteristics who attend their GPs in inner London for cervical smears?

**a** Aged less than 25 years.

**b** African or Afro-Caribbean and aged less than 25 years.

**c** Two or more sexual partners in the previous year.

**d** Condoms not always used.

**e** Presence of mucopurulent discharge.

**f** Friable cervix.

**g** None of the above.

*BMJ.* **316**: 351–2 (survey report)

**4** The prevalence of positive cultures from endocervical and high vaginal swabs in urban UK women (mainly social class 3 in the study sample) with lower genital tract symptoms and normal cervical smears has been found to be as follows.

| | | |
|---|---|---|
| 1. | *Candida albicans* | 17% |
| 2. | *Chlamydia trachomatis* | 12% |
| 3. | *Trichomonas vaginalis* | 3% |
| 4. | *Gonococcus* | 1% |

**a** In the light of these figures, what do you see as the indications for prescribing an antibiotic that will eradicate chlamydia for a woman with vaginitis?

**b** What further information would you like to have in order to make a rational decision?

*Br J Gen Pract.* **41**: 279–81

**5**
a What do you regard as appropriate indications for taking an endocervical swab for chlamydia testing?

b If the result is positive, what do you regard as appropriate management?

*Br J Gen Pract.* **45**: 615–20 (review)

*BMJ.* **307**: 150–1

**6**
In screening for chlamydia, what response rate can be expected in female and male schoolchildren to requests for samples, firstly if samples are to be provided at home and sent to the clinic, and secondly if samples are to be provided at the clinic or GP surgery?

*BMJ.* **316**: 26–7 (survey report)

**7**
Screening for chlamydia.

a According to the government advisory group, which groups should be offered this service?

b What matters remain to be resolved before a government-backed screening programme can be implemented?

*BMJ.* **316**: 1474 (leading article)

**8**
Male partners of women with pelvic inflammatory disease. (*True/False*)

a The majority have urethritis.

b The majority of those with urethritis have no symptoms.

c Treating those with urethritis in a population makes no significant difference to the incidence of salpingitis thereafter.

*BMJ.* **311**: 630 (letter)

**9**
A symptom-free man has been found to have chlamydia on a urethral swab. Under what circumstances would it be worth referring him to the local genitourinary medicine department?

*BMJ.* **314**: 516–17 (letters)

**10**
What seems to be the likeliest means of obtaining a urine sample from the partner of a woman infected with chlamydia?

*BMJ.* **316**: 350–1 (survey report)

**11**
What dose of erythromycin has been found to clear 94% of cervical chlamydia infections – with the failures mainly due to early discontinuation due to gastrointestinal side-effects?

*Br J Gen Pract.* **46**: 255–6 (letter)

**12** A woman has recurring dysuria and frequency, but the mid-stream urine (MSU) shows no abnormalities. What questions or observations might elucidate the cause or yield information that would influence further management? (*List four or more*)

*BMJ.* **303**: 1–2

**13** Genital herpes. (*True/False*)

**a** It is only infective while it is symptomatic.

**b** Viral shedding is likely to be much less frequent with oral acyclovir treatment.

*BMJ.* **314**: 85–6 (editorial)

**14** What means of preventing pelvic inflammatory disease at the time of termination of pregnancy are supported by evidence?

*Br J Gen Pract.* **48**: 1270 (letter)

**15** Sexually transmitted diseases.

**a** What is the drug class of first choice for treating gonorrhoea?

**b** What is the optimal specimen and most sensitive testing technique for chlamydia?

**c** What treatment prevents most recurrences of herpes simplex?

*BMJ.* **316**: 1129–32 (review)

**16** In which part of the world is there currently an epidemic of syphilis?

*BMJ.* **315**: 1018–19 (letter)

# ANSWERS

## Sexual medicine

1  False.

2  Suggestions from the author and from GPs addressing this question were as follows.
   - A teenager's capacity for parenthood and what this implies.
   - The mechanism of fertility and the modes of action of contraceptives.
   - The failure rate of contraceptives and reasons for their failure.
   - The risk of infectious disease as a result of casual sex.
   - Attitudes with regard to respect and responsibility for the opposite sex.
   - The advantages of fidelity.
   - Coping with rejection by a member of the opposite sex.
   - Self-respect and the prevention of abuse.
   - Legal and social restrictions on sexual contact.

3  According to the author, small-group discussion, role play, quizzes and other workshop activities, as well as literature, and encouraging parents to discuss these matters with their children.

4  23.3%.

5  Findings on examination of the blood pressure, peripheral pulses and perineal sensation.
   The following points might be suggested.
   - Erections are easiest in the morning.
   - Discussion of attitude and sexual technique, preferably with the partner.
   - Physical aids – vacuum device.
   - Medicinal aids – sildenafil, alprostadil. Benefit of treating any vitamin E deficiency (treatment of priapism if using medicinal aids).
   - Close control of the diabetes and of serum lipids.

6  a  Oxytocin.
   b  They cause retrograde ejaculation in a proportion of men.
   c  They abolish orgasm independently of ejaculation in up to 20% of users.

7  a  False.
   b  True.
   c  False – they have a neutral effect.

8  a  Thiazides, beta-blockers, antidepressants, metoclopramide, digoxin and cimetidine.

   **b** Do you have spontaneous erections? Can you masturbate?

   **c** Blood pressure, peripheral pulses, bulbocavernous reflex, anal sphincter tone.

   **d** It inhibits phosphodiesterase-5, thus reducing the breakdown of cyclic GMP, the second messenger in the erection reflex.

   **e** Older men in stable relationships.

**9**  **a** One hour before intercourse.

   **b** Headache in 16% of cases, also facial flushing, indigestion, a stuffy nose, and in 3% of cases a temporary bluish tinge to the field of vision.

**10** Instillation into the urethra.

**11**  **a** True – it commonly causes retrograde ejaculation.

   **b** False.

   **c** True – also true of sympathectomy.

**12**  **a** 4 to 5 days.

   **b**  i Probable ovarian failure.

      ii Probable polycystic ovaries.

      iii Consider a dopamine agonist as the first line of treatment.

   **c** Operate to remove the blockage and then provide 6 months of treatment with danazol or a GnRH analogue.

   **d** • Stimulate the ovaries with clomiphene or a similar drug.

      • Remove sperms from plasma of the ejaculate in order to reduce the bacterial content and to concentrate the motile sperms.

      • Time the injection to coincide with ovulation.

   **e** Bilateral tubal blockage.

   **f** On average 20%.

   **g** On average 30%.

**13**  **a** Anxiety and lowered self-esteem, but not usually depression.

   **b** Discuss the process of adjusting to bad news, enlightened attitudes, acceptance of the risk that there will be no children, but the possibility of success using intracytoplasmic sperm injection.

**14**  **a** Varicocoele – found in 25% of cases.

   **b** It is debatable – there is a minimal effect on fertility if surgery is performed after the age of 30 years.

   **c** • Avoid smoking, consuming excess alcohol, and soaking in a hot bath.

      • Avoid nitrofurantoin, tetracycline and colchicine.

      • Hot showers and saunas have no effect on scrotal temperature.

      • Timing intercourse is not of proven benefit.

# Genitourinary medicine

1   a  The premenstrual stage.

   b  Thrush, herpes, allergy, contact sensitivity, psoriasis.

   c  If there is a risk of sexually acquired disease, or if symptoms resist a course of anti-candidal treatment.

   d  Tenderness in the vulva which deters the woman from using a pessary.

   e  This strain may resist treatment with imidazole derivatives, but is usually sensitive to nystatin.

2   a  About 50%.

   b  A reduction of 56% in the incidence of pelvic inflammatory disease.

   c  DNA amplification technique – particularly the ligase chain reaction, performed on urine, vaginal washings obtained using a pipette, or on endocervical and urethral swabs.

   d  It is a single-dose treatment, so there is likely to be better compliance.

3   The prevalence of chlamydial infection in endocervical swabs from women under 35 years of age attending their GPs in inner London for cervical smears was as follows:

   a  aged less than 25 years – 6.0%

   b  African or Afro-Caribbean and aged less than 25 years – 9.1%

   c  two or more sexual partners in the previous year – 7.1%

   d  condoms not always used – 3.5%

   e  presence of mucopurulent discharge – 6.6%

   f  friable cervix – 9.7%

   g  none of the above – 0.8%.

4   a  Doctors answering this question suggested the following indications for treating vaginitis with an anti-chlamydia treatment.

   • Deep dyspareunia, dysmenorrhoea, cervicitis and pain on examination.

   • Recent pregnancy or pelvic surgery.

   • A history of infertility.

   • Non-response to an imidazole.

   b  Further information required for a rational decision includes answers to the following questions.

   • What proportion of vaginal infections are mixed?

   • Can chlamydia be as readily identified on Microtrak if the smear contains other organisms?

   • What proportion of chlamydial infections resolve spontaneously without sequelae?

- What proportion of women with pelvic inflammatory disease previously had symptoms of vaginitis, and what proportion of them received treatment for it?

5 a The author of this review regards screening all fertile women for chlamydial cervicitis as wise if the local prevalence exceeds 6%. Otherwise, women should be screened if they have characteristics that place them in a high-risk group. These include age less than 25 years, being sexually active, using non-barrier methods of contraception, a recent change of partner, having a vaginal discharge, a friable cervix or sterile pyuria, or being about to undergo termination of pregnancy.

 Chlamydial cervicitis appears to meet many of the criteria for screening. It is highly prevalent, it is often asymptomatic, it has serious consequences in some cases and it is readily treatable.

 Screening would be acceptable and practicable if performed at the same time as cervical smears. Furthermore, women with multiple sexual partners are a high-risk group, although these women may also be least likely to comply with screening. However, we remain uncertain about the natural history of the condition, the rate of recurrence after treatment, the predictive validity of the test, and the implications of a positive screening result for tubal infertility and problems during pregnancy. Alternatives, such as a public awareness programme about the dangers of promiscuity without condoms and of untreated vaginal and pelvic infections, may be more cost-effective than screening. Since testing would be more expensive than treatment, the alternative policy of blind treatment of suspect cases also needs to be considered.

 b Appropriate management of a positive result consists of prescribing doxycycline 100 mg bd for 7 days, or for 14 days if there is pelvic pain. In addition, sexual partners should be treated, and both partners should have follow-up samples checked for infection.

6

|  | Males | Females |
| --- | --- | --- |
| Home sampling (%) | 34 | 48 |
| Sampling at clinic or GP surgery (%) | 19 | 38 |

7 a Men and women with relevant symptoms, women attending genitourinary medicine clinics and for terminations of pregnancy, sexually active women aged under 25 years, and women aged over 25 years who have changed partner during the previous 12 months.

 b The costs and benefits of different approaches, the need for public and professional education, the acceptability of screening, which tests, specimens and treatments to use, and the most effective way of tracing and testing partners.

8 a True – 30 of 34 cases in one survey, 46 of 58 cases in another, and 117 of 200 cases in yet another.

 b True 36 of 46 cases in one survey, and 96 of 117 cases in another.

 c False – in Sweden the incidence of salpingitis fell by 40% over a period of 10 years when a policy was introduced of treating male partners of women with pelvic inflammatory disease who themselves showed evidence of urethritis.

9 Chlamydial infection in a man is often asymptomatic. It is readily treated in general practice. The condition is non-problematic for the man, but may pose future problems for sexual partners. It may also be associated with other genital infections, although it would be unusual for these to be asymptomatic. We are taught to send all sexually acquired infections to the department of genitourinary medicine for accurate and complete diagnosis and contact tracing. However, most GPs answering this question thought that they would be happy to treat the man without further investigation, and to advise him that his partner should be investigated. Only if the man had multiple sexual partners would a referral to the genitourinary medicine clinic be justified.

10 Give the woman a sample bottle and request form and ask her to suggest to her partner that he provides an early-morning sample. Inviting the male partner to visit his doctor had a much lower response rate (28% compared to 68%).

11 Erythromycin 500 mg bd for 10 days.

12 • Is the dysuria internal (cystitis) or external (urethritis, vulval irritation)?
   • Is there a good stream of urine? If not, residual urine may be a contributory factor.
   • Is there stress incontinence or urge incontinence?
   • What toilet preparations are being used? Contact sensitivity may be contributing.
   • Does the cystitis coincide with sexual activity or a phase of the menstrual cycle?
   • Is there any evidence of marital disharmony?
   • Is the vaginal mucosa atrophic?
   • Check the urine pH and concentration.
   • Swab for chlamydia.

13 a False – 70% of transmissions occur during periods of presumed subclinical viral shedding. Females are more at risk of contracting the infection from a single episode of sexual intercourse with an infected partner than are males.
   b True – viral shedding was detectable in 5.8% of patient-days in patients on placebo but in only 0.4% of patient-days in patients on acyclovir.

14 • Screening for genital infections and treating those who are positive.
   • Universal antibiotic cover at the time of the termination.

15 a Fluoroquinolones – but resistant strains are appearing.
   b Ligase chain reaction on genital swabs.
   c Long-term continuous treatment with acyclovir 40 mg bd is indicated if there are more than six recurrences per year.

16 The former USSR.

# SPORTS MEDICINE

**1** Prescribing for sportsmen.

   **a** Which drugs that GPs commonly prescribe may be taken in all innocence by sportsmen and later cause them to be debarred from an event?

   **b** Which drugs might a sportsman seek to obtain on a GP prescription with a view to improving his performance in a competitive event? (*10 points*)

*BMJ.* **313**: 211–15 (review article)

**2** Which classes of medicines increase the risk of heatstroke?

*BMJ.* **315**: 556 (citation)

**3** Jumper's knee.

   **a** What are the clinical features?

   **b** What investigation will clinch the diagnosis?

*BMJ.* **316**: 320 (citation)

**4** At what risks do sportsmen who use anabolic steroids put themselves? (*4 points*)

*BMJ.* **313**: 100–1 (case reports)

**5** An adult with a history of excessive sweating and heat exhaustion on strenuous exercise in a hot climate has been found to have an abnormally high sweat sodium and to carry mutations for cystic fibrosis genes. What implications does this have for routine practice? (*2 or more points*)

*BMJ.* **310**: 579–80

# ANSWERS

1  a Pseudoephedrine, phenylpropanolamine, dextropropoxyphene and intra-articular steroids.

   b Dextropropoxyphene, beta-blockers, diuretics, erythropoietin, probenecid, intra-articular steroids.

2  Neuroleptics and anticholinergics.

3  a The clinical features of jumper's knee are pain at the front of the knee and tenderness of the patellar tendon near its patellar attachment.

   b Ultrasound scan will show a hyperechoic region at the inferior margin of the patella. The condition is common in basketball players and footballers, as well as in jumpers. It may last over a year, and one-third of cases require surgery.

4  They put themselves at risk of hypogonadotrophic hypogonadism, altered lipid concentrations, liver disease, gynaecomastia, reduced libido, mood changes, dependence, withdrawal effects and prostatic carcinoma.

5  The *British Medical Journal* presented a case history of a soldier who developed heatstroke after running in hot climates, and who was subsequently found to have high sweat sodium and chloride levels and to carry two of the eight mutations associated with cystic fibrosis. He was azoospermic, but lung and pancreas function were normal. GPs addressing this question suggested that this might have the following implications for routine practice.

   • Patients with cystic fibrosis may need to be reminded of the need to avoid outdoor exercise in hot weather, and to drink isotonic fluid in large quantities if exposed to warmth.

   • Patients with heat exhaustion should have their electrolytes checked, and if they are abnormal then appropriate replacement therapy is indicated. Men with heat exhaustion and abnormally low serum sodium and chloride levels under minimal provocation may undergo sweat analysis and semen analysis and be advised thereafter.

   • Genetic counselling may be indicated for patients who are found to have the abnormal gene, but on the basis of this evidence it would appear unlikely that they would produce a child severely handicapped by cystic fibrosis.

# SURGERY

## General practice and out-patient surgery

**1** Guidelines recommend the following arrangement for GPs undertaking minor surgery. Do you think that they are essential for a GP excising a sebaceous cyst on practice premises? If not, state a reason for your view.

**a** The couch to be in the middle of the operating room.

**b** A mobile light.

**c** A plastic airway.

**d** A readily available, in-date vial of adrenaline.

**e** An autoclave or dry-heat sterilizer.

**f** Sterile gloves.

**g** Sterile drapes and clips.

**h** A mask for the surgeon.

**i** A third person within hailing distance in the building.

*BMJ.* **302**: 941–2

**2** You are preparing to lance an abscess for a drug addict of uncertain sexual habits. What extra precautions will you take to minimize the risk of a viral infection? (*3 points*)

*BMJ.* **305**: 1337–42

**3** What technique will reduce leakage of a drug injected intramuscularly?

*BMJ.* **311**: 1368 (letter)

**4** Tap water is as safe as sterile saline for irrigating dirty wounds. (*True/False*)

*BMJ.* **314**: 1702 (citation)

**5** Feet.

    **a** What features differentiate a plantar corn from a wart? (*6 points*)

    **b** How would you know where to position a pad in the sole of a shoe in order to avoid pressure on a callosity under a metatarsal head?

    *BMJ.* **312**: 1405 (review)

**6** How might a GP with facilities for surgery under local anaesthetic treat a small pilonidal sinus?

    *BMJ.* **305**: 410–12

**7** How might you treat a patient with a pre-tibial laceration that has raised a flap of skin? (*3 points*)

    *Br J Gen Pract.* **93**: 174

**8** What are the particular benefits and dangers of the following methods of treatment of haemorrhoids? (*8 or more points*)

    **a** Injection of sclerosant above the pectinate line.

    **b** Ligation banding.

    **c** Infra-red coagulation.

    *BMJ.* **314**: 1211–12 (leading article)

**9** In sclerotherapy for haemorrhoids, what clinical features indicate that the injection is being given correctly into the submucosa? (*2 points*)

    *BMJ.* **314**: 419 (case reports)

# In-patient surgery

**1** List three physical examination techniques to elicit peritonism. (*3 points*)

    *BMJ.* **308**: 1336

    *BMJ.* **309**: 1192

**2** The following may be presenting features of an abdominal aneurysm: (*True/False*)

    **a** pain in the groin

    **b** back pain

    **c** intermittent claudication

d  bloody diarrhoea

e  palpable enlargement of a kidney

f  raised venous pressure.

*BMJ.* **303**:1127–9

---

**3**  Lumps in the neck. (*True/False*)

a  Branchial cysts are usually found in infants.

b  A thyroglossal cyst will move on swallowing.

c  A dermoid cyst may extend under the skull.

d  Cystic hygromas can be transilluminated.

e  Cat-scratch fever is due to a virus.

f  Avian TB causes a positive Mantoux test.

*BMJ.* **312**: 368–71 (review)

---

**4**  A patient in pain with suspected appendicitis should be given an analgesic before being sent to hospital. (*True/False*)

*BMJ.* **305**: 554–6, 1020

---

**5**  What advice on oral intake is advisable for healthy patients who are free of nausea or shock, and not taking drugs that delay gastric emptying, but who are likely to require an anaesthetic within the next few hours?

*BMJ.* **314**: 162 (leading article)

---

**6**  Paediatric surgery. (*True/False*)

a  An inguinal hernia in a baby should be left until the baby is 1 year old before it is repaired.

b  A hydrocele in an infant boy requires no surgical treatment.

c  A fully descended testis in a 5-year-old boy will always remain descended thereafter.

d  Ultrasound is reliable for locating an impalpable testis.

*BMJ.* **312**: 564–7 (review)

---

**7**  Brachial plexus neuropathy after radiotherapy can be treated surgically. (*True/False*)

*BMJ.* **312**: 780 (letter)

---

**8**  Hernia. (*True/False*)

a  Inguinal hernias have a higher rate of complication than femoral hernias.

**b** Trusses for hernias have no significant risk of adverse effect.

*BMJ.* **301**: 1319

**9** Gallstones. (*True/False*)

**a** Ultrasound is reliable for detecting stones in the common bile duct.

**b** Shock-wave lithotripsy is best used together with oral bile salt treatment.

**c** Cholecystectomy is likely to cure coexisting heartburn.

**d** Post-cholecystectomy diarrhoea is usually a permanent problem.

*BMJ.* **311**: 99–104

**10** How soon after a laparoscopic cholecystectomy is the patient likely to go home?

*BMJ.* **302**: 303–4

**11** What proportion of patients who undergo cholecystectomy continue to experience pain thereafter?

*BMJ.* **306**: 1688

**12** How soon after an uncomplicated operation may an office-worker with no significant postoperative pain return to work?

*BMJ.* **309**: 216–17

**13** How soon after herniorrhaphy do patients usually return to sedentary work if the operation is performed by the following techniques:

**a** open-mesh repair

**b** laparoscopic surgery?

*BMJ.* **316**: 103–10

**14** Advances in surgery.

**a** What drugs are useful for preventing postoperative nausea? (*4 points*)

**b** What local anaesthetic technique reduces postoperative pain after a laparotomy? (*1 point*)

**c** What operation seems to be useful for controlling gastro-oesophageal reflux? (*1 point*)

*BMJ.* **315**: 586–9 (review)

**15** Prioritizing patients on waiting-lists for elective surgery.

**a** How would you weigh up the relative importance of objective physical observations, morbidity, functional observations, and patients' reports of the influence of the condition on their lives? (*3 or more points*)

**b** Are there any other factors worthy of consideration in this context?

*BMJ.* **314**: 131–8 (education and debate)

**16** Plastic surgeons can remove scars. (*True/False*)

*BMJ.* **314**: 991 (leading article)

**17** Which vital sign is likely to be affected first when a fit young person suffers internal haemorrhage?

*BMJ.* **314**: 1549 (case report)

# ANSWERS

## General practice and out-patient surgery

1   The consensus from GPs addressing this question was as follows.

   **a** The couch in the middle of the operating room – not essential, as minor operations do not require an assistant working from the other side of the body.

   **b** A mobile light – essential.

   **c** Airway – essential, and cheap and easy to obtain.

   **d** A readily available, in-date vial of adrenalin – essential.

   **e** An autoclave or dry-heat sterilizer – not essential but highly desirable. Sterilization by immersion or boiling is also acceptable, and many practices obtain all of their surgery packs from the local central sterile-supply department.

   **f** Sterile gloves – essential.

   **g** Sterile drapes and clips – not essential, but skin-cleansing solution is essential.

   **h** A mask for the surgeon – essential.

   **i** A third person within hailing distance in the building – highly desirable, in case there is something missing from the trolley, or to answer the telephone, as well as to deal with problems arising as a result of the procedure.

2   Operating on a patient who may be a carrier of hepatitis B requires particular caution. Members suggested avoiding surgery if at all possible, and checking the patient's HBsAg status before operating. The attendants should be immunized against hepatitis B. Prior to the operation, inessential equipment should be removed from the area of the operation. If attendants have any broken skin it should be dressed. The operator and attendants may wear double gloves and impervious gowns, masks and goggles. Sharp objects should be placed in disinfectant after use as a preliminary to sterilization, and needles should be put in the incinerator bin without resheathing. Spillages should be wiped up immediately and the area wiped with disinfectant after the procedure. Samples for the laboratory may need to be labelled 'Infection Risk'. An extractor fan would be a wise investment if such procedures are commonplace.

3   Z-track – push the needle in a little, move it sideways, and then advance it before injecting.

4   True.

5   **a** • Warts have rapid onset, whereas corns develop over weeks, months or years.

     • Warts may or may not be under bony prominences, whereas corns always are.

     • Skin lines pass around warts but through corns.

- Warts are painful on squeezing from side to side, whereas corns are painful on direct pressure.
- End arteries of warts are visible on paring, but are not visible in corns.
- Warts recur rapidly after shaving and padding, but corns recur more slowly – at least a week after shaving.

b  Apply lipstick to the callosity and see where it leaves a mark on the sole of the shoe. The pad with a hole in the middle should be positioned around this point.

6  Shave the area. Either curette the sinus, but aim to avoid a midline scar, or apply phenol for 1 min and repeat this procedure twice, separated by intervals of 1 min. Then follow up with weekly observation and shaving for several weeks.

7  The author suggests cutting the loose flap of skin, scraping off the underlying fat and using it in patches for grafting. In many cases it may suffice to clean the flap with sterile saline, stretch it over the denuded area and secure it with a non-adherent dressing.

8  a  Risk of causing impotence, and difficulty of placing the sclerosant correctly.

b  This requires two people – one to hold the anoscope and the other to use the ligator. It can be very painful if the band is applied too low, and it has been associated with sepsis.

c  This method is usually quick and painless, but may require multiple visits. It is the best of the three methods listed in a recent clinical trial, with 80% of patients being symptom free at 3 months.

9  Striation appearing at the injection site, and the absence of pain.

## In-patient surgery

1  • Check by percussion for rebound tenderness.
   • Check for localized abdominal pain provoked by coughing.
   • Check by having the patient tense and relax the abdominal wall.

2  a  True.
   b  True.
   c  True.
   d  True.
   e  True.
   f  True.

3  a  False – they are usually found in adolescents or adults.
   b  True – there is a midline swelling which moves on tongue protrusion or swallowing. It is prone to infection.
   c  True – therefore a sebum-secreting swelling under the chin, at the nasal bridge or

between the lateral border of the eye and the hairline which appears to extend to the bone should be examined by skull X-ray or CT scan.

d  True.

e  False – it is due to a bacterium, *Rochamilaea henselae*. Usually a papule is present at the inoculation site and tender lymphadenopathy appears about 2 weeks after the scratch. Diagnosis is by aspiration and use of a Warthin-Starry silver stain, or by node excision.

f  False – but it requires surgical excision of affected lymph nodes and any chronic sinus or skin.

4  True.

5  Solids should be stopped at least 4 h before the anaesthetic, but clear fluids may be taken up to 2 h before the anaesthetic. Used in this way, they appear to reduce the volume and increase the pH of the gastric fluid aspirated at the time of the anaesthetic.

6  a  False – it should be treated as soon as the baby's condition permits, as there is a high rate of complications.

b  True – 90% of cases will subside spontaneously.

c  False – occasionally descended but retractile testes can reascend after the age of 5 years, and require orchidopexy.

d  False – ultrasound and CT are both insensitive in young children.

7  True.

8  a  False – femoral hernias are more likely to strangulate.

b  False – they may enlarge the hernial orifice, and may cause adhesions within the sac, or adhesion of the spermatic cord to the hernial sac. They also increase the risk of strangulation.

9  a  False – these stones may be difficult to detect as they may be obscured by gas in the duodenum.

b  True – after fragmentation of stones with shock waves, oral dissolution treatment prevents them from reforming.

c  False – cholecystectomy may exacerbate heartburn because of bile gastritis.

d  False – post-cholecystectomy diarrhoea usually resolves without treatment.

10  2 days.

11  20–30%.

12  Within 1 week.

13  a  Open-mesh repair – 14–18 days.

b  Laparoscopic surgery – 10–11 days.

14  a  Using propofol as an anaesthetic, intra-operative use of antinauseants such as ondansetron, and postoperative use of a combination of droperidol and metoclopramide.

**b** Injecting bupivacaine into the incision site before the operation.

**c** Fundoplication.

15 **a** In the absence of a scoring system, patients waiting for non-urgent elective surgery are all accorded similar priority. However, those who exaggerate their symptoms and pester the surgical department personally or through their GPs may obtain earlier treatment than is fair.

A scoring system is not a complete answer to the problem, as patients may still exaggerate their symptoms in order to get a higher priority score. However, in New Zealand the adoption of such scoring systems – one for each major procedure – led to the government releasing more cash to deal with waiting-lists. At least one health authority is seeking to develop a similar system here.

Objective physical observations reflecting the likely benefit from surgery deserve high priority in such a scoring system. Physical observations on comorbidity which might affect the duration or degree of practical benefit obtained from the procedure are also objective and should be given high weighting. If the operation will affect the patient's requirement for social care, this also merits a place in the scoring system.

Symptom severity and functional ability may best be gauged by the GP when patients first present and before they are fully aware of how this may affect the waiting period. One may also ask about symptom severity in several different ways, or on two or more occasions, and check for consistency in the patient's answers.

**b** GPs addressing this question also suggested the following further observations that could be useful: the patient's ability to have the surgery performed privately; the dangers of the procedure in the patient's current state of health; and the patient's willingness to adopt health-seeking behaviour in order to maximize the benefits obtained from the procedure.

16 False – for affected people, counselling support is a better approach.

17 Respiratory rate.

# TESTS

**1** Why might immediate availability of results for the following tests be useful to general practitioners?

**a** C-reactive protein.

**b** Cardiac troponin T.

*BMJ.* **312**: 263–4 (leading article), 1049–50 (leading article)

**2** A chronically high level of C-reactive protein is predictive of which future disorders?

*BMJ.* **314**: 1210 (citations)

**3** Storing whole blood at a relatively high ambient temperature for a period of 4 h is likely to cause a rise in serum potassium concentration. (*True/False*)

*BMJ.* **312**: 1652–4 (research report)

*BMJ.* **314**: 1210 (citations)

**4** Ankle systolic blood pressure can be measured with an ultrasound fetal heart monitor. (*True/False*)

*BMJ.* **313**: 1440–3 (research report)

**5** Magnetic resonance imaging is the best available technique for showing the following: (*True/False*)

**a** acute cerebral haemorrhage

**b** cerebral oedema

**c** a cerebrovascular malformation

**d** a cerebral tumour

**e** lumbar disc herniation

**f** avascular necrosis of bone

**g** a torn ligament in the knee

**h** a renal tumour.

*BMJ.* **303**: 105–9

**6** Uses of nuclear medicine.

**a** How much bone matrix needs to be lost before the loss is apparent on an X-ray?

**b** Bone scintigrams using radioactive biphosphonates may be useful to demonstrate what conditions? (*10 points*)

**c** What property of 99mTc DMSA makes it the best means of demonstrating a renal scar?

**d** What advantage does a scintimammogram have over a conventional mammogram?

**e** What isotope can be used to treat painful bony metastases?

*BMJ.* **316**: 1140–6 (review)

# ANSWERS

1    a   To differentiate between viral and bacterial causes of a chest infection, and to differentiate between serious and trivial acute abdominal pain.

     a and b   To determine whether recent onset of angina justifies admission for anticoagulation.

2    Heart attack and stroke.

3    False – in the first few hours the effect of storing blood at a relatively high temperature is to cause a small fall in the serum potassium concentration. Thereafter serum potassium levels will rise due to haemolysis.

4    True – although manufacturers usually recommend a detector with a higher waveband.

5    a   False.

     b   True.

     c   True.

     d   True.

     e   True.

     f   True.

     g   True.

     h   False.

6    a   50%.

     b   Primary tumours, metastases, stress fractures, shin splints, avascular necrosis of hips or knees, to differentiate between loosening and infection of joint prostheses, to diagnose metabolic bone disease, to perform a joint survey on arthritis, and to investigate bone pain of unknown origin.

     c   It is extracted by tubular cells.

     d   It has greater specificity, particularly in radiologically dense breasts (its negative predictive value is 97%, so it reduces the number of biopsies required).

     e   Strontium 89 relieves pain in 75% of cases, typically 1–3 weeks after treatment.

# UROLOGY

**1** Urology. (*True/False*)

**a** Haematospermia justifies immediate investigation.

**b** Blood in the urine restricted to the initial flow of urine in an elderly man is suggestive of prostatic carcinoma.

*BMJ.* **312**: 1032–4 (review)

**2** What laboratory observation may differentiate red cells of glomerular origin in the urine from red cells from lower in the urinary tract? What techniques are suitable for this observation? (*3 points*)

*BMJ.* **309**: 70–2

**3** A patient has had renal colic on three occasions and produced a stone on one, but subsequently lost it. What investigations are justified to test for a metabolic abnormality? (*8 points*)

*BMJ.* **312**: 1219–21

**4** Ultrasound of the renal tract: (*True/False*)

**a** is more likely than IVP to detect a stone in the kidney

**b** is more likely than IVP to detect a stone in the ureter

**c** is more likely than IVP to detect a stone in the bladder

**d** can be used to quantify residual urine.

*BMJ.* **313**: 1079 (letter)

**5** Testicular torsion. (*5 points*)

**a** What clinical pointers may help to differentiate epididymitis from torsion?

**b** What investigation other than a surgical one may permit a positive diagnosis?

**c** What late complication may follow fixation?

*BMJ.* **312**: 435–7 (review)

**6** Erectile impotence.
  **a** What is the prevalence at age 40 years, and at age 65 years?
  **b** What question(s) would be useful in screening for an endocrine cause?
  **c** Which antihypertensives appear to be neutral in their effect on the problem?
  **d** A man who used a papaverine injection to get an erection 4 h ago still has an erect penis. What should he do?

  *BMJ.* **309**: 957–60 (review)

  *BMJ.* **312**: 838–40 (review)

**7** List the urinary symptoms that are common in middle-aged and elderly men in descending order of their prevalence to a degree that is bothersome. (*7 points*)

  *Br J Gen Pract.* **46**: 349–52

**8** What symptoms are most suggestive of bladder outlet obstruction? (*3 points*)

  *BMJ.* **309**: 929–30

**9** What form of monitoring may differentiate between urinary frequency due to a bladder or prostate disorder and frequency due to high fluid intake? (*1 point*)

  *BMJ.* **307**: 1057

**10** Which men with prostatic hypertrophy but a normal or only slightly raised prostate-specific antigen (PSA) justify referral to a urologist? (*2 or more points*)

  *Br J Gen Pract.* **94**: 499–502 (research report)

  *BMJ.* **310**: 202 (citation)

**11** If there are symptoms of urinary outflow obstruction and an enlarged prostate, the following are strong indications for prostatectomy: (*True/False*)
  **a** residual volume of 200 mL
  **b** elevated creatinine or urea
  **c** haematuria.

  *BMJ.* **314**: 1215–16 (leading article)

  *Br J Gen Pract.* **97**: 235–8 (review)

**12** What suggestions on self-management of the condition would you make to a man with moderate symptoms of urinary obstruction who typically voids about 170 mL at a time and who has no features of prostatic cancer? (*2 or more points*)

  *BMJ.* **310**: 1113–17

**13** Symptoms of prostatic hypertrophy are bound to get worse. (*True/False*)

*BMJ.* **307**: 201

**14** From the results of this study, what is the risk of acute retention if patients who may merit surgery for benign prostatic hyperplasia are randomized to a policy of watchful waiting for the next 5 years?

*BMJ.* **316**: 154 (citation)

**15** What two types of drug may provide relief for a man with benign prostatic hypertrophy?

*BMJ.* **304**: 1198–9

**16** Drug treatment for benign prostatic hyperplasia. (*True/False*)

**a** Terazosin can be expected to alleviate all symptoms within a few weeks.

**b** Terazosin can be expected to improve the urine flow rate.

**c** Finasteride can be expected to reduce symptoms markedly within 1 year.

**d** Finasteride can be expected to increase flow rates within a few weeks.

**e** 5-alpha-reductase inhibitors may reduce potency and ability to ejaculate.

*BMJ.* **314**: 1215–16 (leading article)

*Br J Gen Pract.* **97**: 235–8 (review)

**17** An old man with benign prostatic hypertrophy is too frail for a TURP. What other medical or surgical treatments may relieve his urinary retention? (*4 points*)

*BMJ.* **309**: 716–18

**18** Prostate-specific antigen. (*True/False*)

**a** Levels of more than 20 mg/L PSA make it almost certain that there is prostatic cancer with metastatic spread.

**b** Taking gland volume into account provides a better means of discriminating between benign hypertrophy and cancer.

*BMJ.* **308**: 780–2

**19** From the results of this study, what level of PSA in a man aged 60–74 years would indicate an even chance of developing prostatic cancer over the next 3 years?

*BMJ.* **311**: 1340–3 (research report)

**20** Prostatic serum antigen values are affected by the following: (*True/False*)

a acute retention

b catheterization

c prostatitis

d digital rectal examination.

*BMJ.* **312**: 767–70 (review)

**21** What effect does taking finasteride have on plasma PSA levels?

*BMJ.* **315**: 371 (letter)

**22** A man with mild urinary obstruction symptoms has a raised PSA level. What investigations should follow?

*BMJ.* **304**: 1198–9

**23** Screening for prostate cancer.

a What reduction in death rate from prostate cancer has been found in a large American trial of screening men aged 45–80 years by PSA and rectal examination, followed by ultrasound for suspect cases?

b What was the cost per case identified?

c Which demographic group in the USA is believed to be at increased risk of prostate cancer?

*BMJ.* **316**: 1626 (news item)

**24** Prostatic cancer.

a By how much is a man's life likely to be shortened if he has a moderately well-differentiated prostatic cancer?

b What proportion of men dying of prostatic cancer are under 75 years of age?

*BMJ.* **316**: 1903–4 (letters)

**25** There is insufficient evidence on which to base advice on optimal treatment for men with early prostatic carcinoma. However, what considerations should be discussed with them in helping them to reach a decision? (*5 or more points*)

*BMJ.* **316**: 1919–20 (editorial)

**26** What mortality is associated with transrectal ultrasound and biopsy?

*BMJ.* **315**:1549–50 (personal view)

**27** Bladder cancer may present with symptoms other than haematuria. What are they? (*2 points*)

*BMJ.* **308**: 910–13

**28** A 70-year-old man has come home after a laparotomy but still requires di-hydrocodeine to control his pain. He develops urinary retention and you are called in the late evening. In this situation the following measures can be recommended. (*True/False*)

**a** Insert an indwelling urethral catheter.

**b** Insert a temporary urethral catheter and train the patient in self-catheterization.

**c** Request that a suprapubic catheter be inserted.

**d** Prescribe a tricyclic antidepressant as an adjunct to pain control and reduce intake of dihydrocodeine.

**e** Prescribe indoramine.

*BMJ.* **302**: 864S

**29** An elderly man with nocturnal incontinence has an enlarged prostate and a palpably dilated but non-tender bladder, and is unfit for major surgery. How should he be catheterized?

*BMJ.* **312**: 838–40 (review)

**30** Intermittent self-catheterization for patients with neuropathic bladder. (*True/False*)

**a** It can prevent renal damage.

**b** If the volume of residual urine is less than 50–100 mL, intermittent catheterization is unlikely to be helpful.

**c** Strict aseptic technique is required.

**d** Catheters may best be stored in a dilute solution of sodium hypochlorite.

**e** Vaseline is useful for lubricating the passage of the catheter.

*BMJ.* **312**: 103–7 (review)

**31** What insidious side-effect is associated with the use of oxybutinin but is reversible on withdrawal?

*BMJ.* **315**: 1363–4

# ANSWERS

1 a False – it is usually attributed to non-specific prostatitis and subsides spontaneously.

   b True.

2 Dysmorphic red cells identified on phase-contrast microscopy or by Coulter-counter analysis are likely to be of glomerular origin.

3 • Serum calcium, phosphate and uric acid.

   • 24-h urine pH and concentrations of oxalate, calcium, phosphate and uric acid, spot urine test for cystine.

4 a True.

   b False.

   c True.

   d True.

5 a Pyuria, dysuria or urethral discharge.

   b Ultrasound.

   c Testicular atrophy.

6 a 2% at age 40 years, 25–30% at age 65 years.

   b Erectile impotence may be classified as psychogenic, endocrine, neural or vascular. Screening questions may help the doctor to decide which avenue to pursue. Low levels of androgen or raised levels of prolactin are reflected early on in a loss of libido, so if the desire for sexual contact or arousal is as strong as ever, these disorders may be put at the bottom of the list. We are familiar with the questions and measurements used to screen for diabetes, the other common endocrine cause of impotence. It also seems useful to ask whether erections are normal during masturbation but difficult to obtain when with a partner, as this would suggest a psychogenic component.

   c Calcium antagonists and ACE inhibitors.

   d • Walk up and down the stairs in order to channel more blood flow to the legs.

     • Apply ice to the penis.

     • If these measures fail, drain off 20–40 mL of blood from the penis via a needle applied laterally, and inject 10 mL of dilute phenylephrine or noradrenaline.

7 From the results of this survey:

   • urgency, 20%

   • dribbling, 19%

- nocturia (twice or more), 16.5%
- incomplete emptying, 10.5%
- weak urinary stream, 9.5%
- intermittency, 8%
- straining, 4.5%.

8 Hesitancy, poor stream, and a feeling of fullness at the end of micturition.

9 A frequency–volume chart of urinary output.

10 Those with symptoms that frequently intrude upon their lives and/or who are repeatedly unable to pass 150 mL urine.

11 a True.
  b True.
  c True.

12 Reduce fluid intake in the evening. Limit intake of alcohol and caffeine-containing drinks. Try to resist the urge to empty the bladder until it is full, using pelvic floor exercises to weaken the urge. Void as completely as you can, aiming to produce more than 150 mL each time.

13 False – in a substantial proportion of cases they remit, at least temporarily.

14 2% per annum. One-third of these patients came to surgery.

15 Alpha-blockers and testosterone 5–alpha-reductase inhibitor.

16 a False – symptom scores fell by 32–44% in patients on terazosin and by 23% in controls.
  b True – in patients with an initial flow rate averaging 10.5 mL/s, there was an improvement of 2.7 mL/s on terazosin and 1.4 mL/s on placebo.
  c False – in patients with average symptom scores of 16, there was a decrease of 2.6 on placebo and 3.2 on terazosin.
  d False – in patients with an initial flow rate averaging 10.5 mL/s, there was an improvement of 1.6 mL/s on finasteride and 1.4 mL/s on placebo.
  e True.

17 Alpha-blockers (moderately), 5-alpha-reductase inhibitor (slowly and slightly), microwave thermotherapy, laser ablation, ultrasound.

18 a False – however, 60 mg/L is strongly predictive of metastatic disease.
  b True.

19 Twelve times the normal median level.

20 a True.
  b True.
  c True.
  d False.

21 It halves PSA levels after about 6 months.

22 Rectal examination, transrectal ultrasound, repeat PSA, urine flow studies.

23 a In the screened population the mortality was 15/100 000, compared to 48/100 000 in controls.

b $3000 – well below the cost per case identified for screening for cervical or breast cancer.

c Black Americans.

24 a If the cancer is moderately differentiated, as 75% of them are, the average loss of life duration is 4–5 years. If the cancer is undifferentiated, the average figure is 7–8 years.

b About 50%.

25 How well differentiated the cancer is, life expectancy in the absence of cancer, risks of incontinence and impotence after surgery, effects of radiotherapy, effects of androgen deprivation, new therapies (cryotherapy and brachytherapy), the possibility of entering a clinical trial, and the patient's own attitudes to balancing immediate side-effects against the prospect of a long-term increase in life expectancy.

26 0.4% or 1 in 250.

27 Pelvic pain and recurrent urine infection.

28 a True – inserting an indwelling catheter would provide sure control of what would probably only be a temporary problem.

b False – only the most stoical patient could be expected to learn to use the technique of intermittent self-catheterization in the middle of the night.

c False – the catheter would probably only be required temporarily, as the dihydrocodeine is likely to have precipitated the problem, so a suprapubic catheter would be inappropriate.

d False – a tricyclic antidepressant would probably aggravate the urinary retention.

e True – indoramin or another alpha-blocker could be prescribed before the catheter is withdrawn to ease the flow of urine thereafter. All such patients would require a referral to the local urologist, but an emergency night-time visit to casualty could be avoided in most cases.

29 A suprapubic catheter would be better than a transurethral catheter, so that trials without a catheter can be conducted simply by clamping the catheter.

30 a True – untreated neuropathic bladder commonly leads to vesico-ureteric reflux and ascending infections.

b True – this implies that the bladder is still contractile or that the sphincter is so weak that intermittent catheterization will not prevent incontinence.

c False – clean technique is all that should be expected of patients who have to use the technique many times a day.

d True.

e False – water-based gel is better.

31 Cognitive dysfunction.

# VENOUS THROMBOSIS AND VENOUS ULCERS

## Diagnosis

**1**   Occlusion of superficial veins with a tourniquet below the knee is likely to cause pain on walking if a DVT is present. (*True/False*)

*BMJ.* **303**: 1462–5

*BMJ.* **304**: 107–10

**2**   What blood test currently seems useful to exclude a possible diagnosis of recent-onset DVT or pulmonary embolism?

*BMJ.* **309**: 1525–6 (editorial)

**3**   A patient, previously well, who develops a DVT is at significantly increased risk of cancer. (*True/False*)

*BMJ.* **316**: 1544 (citation)

**4**   What laboratory results would help to differentiate rhabdomyolysis from a DVT in a patient with a swollen calf? (*5 or more points*)

*BMJ.* **309**: 1361–2 (case reports)

**5**   An immobile patient develops breathlessness and chest pain suggestive of pulmonary embolism. He has no symptoms or signs in his legs. What inference can you draw if a Doppler ultrasound study of his leg veins is negative?

*BMJ.* **314**: 4265–9 (review)

**6**   What percentage of 'venous' ulcers are likely to be reclassified as probably unsuitable for treatment with compression on the basis of Doppler ultrasound measurement of ankle and arm systolic blood pressure?

*BMJ.* **303**: 776–9

**7** What investigation may determine whether a patient with a leg ulcer may benefit from surgery to his or her superficial veins?

*BMJ.* **313**: 943 (letter)

**8** Venous ulcers.

a When a venous ulcer is first diagnosed, what investigations are needed to direct treatment? (*2 points*)

b What proportion of sufferers can benefit from venous surgery?

c What proportion of sufferers have coexisting arterial disease?

*BMJ.* **316**: 407–8 (leading article)

**9** Ankle systolic blood pressure can be measured with an ultrasound fetal heart monitor. (*True/False*)

*BMJ.* **313**: 1440–3 (research report)

# Management

**1** What three simple measures may prevent formation or extension of a calf-vein DVT in a bedridden elderly patient?

*BMJ.* **303**: 1260–2

**2** Anti-platelet treatment to prevent DVT and pulmonary embolism. (*True/False*)

a It appears to be effective for medical patients who are immobilized for long periods.

b Aspirin is contraindicated if subcutaneous heparin is also used.

*BMJ.* **308**: 235–44

**3** Wearing compression stockings for 2 years after a DVT reduces the risk of post-thrombotic pain. What is the prevalence of the pain 2 years after the DVT:

a in those who do not wear compression stockings

b in those who do?

*BMJ.* **314**: 849 (news report)

**4** Having a factor V Leiden and a history of DVT justifies lifelong anticoagulation. (*True/False*)

*BMJ.* **316**: 95–9 (research report)

**5** Compression helps most venous ulcers to heal. What refinements to the technique of compression bandaging appear to add to the benefits? (*2 points*)

*BMJ.* **315**: 576–9

**6** What median healing times should one expect for leg ulcers treated by the following methods:

**a** four-layer compression bandaging at a weekly clinic

**b** routine dressing by district nurses?

*BMJ.* **316**: 1487–91 (trial report)

**7** Venous insufficiency and leg ulcers.

**a** What surgical technique, applied early in the course of the disease, holds most promise of preventing its progress?

**b** What topical applications to the ulcer are currently favoured? (*3 points*)

**c** What grafting operations may speed the healing of an ulcer? (*2 points*)

*BMJ.* **314**: 1019–22 (review)

**8** Hyperbaric oxygen for venous ulcers.

**a** What difference in healing rate has been shown with this treatment?

**b** What may be its mechanisms of action?

*BMJ.* **315**: 188–9 (letters)

# ANSWERS

## Diagnosis

1 True.

2 D-Dimer.

3 False – in a case–control study of 15 348 patients with DVT, 1737 patients later developed cancer, compared to the 1372 expected. The increased risk was not statistically significant.

4 Dipstick haematuria in the absence of erythrocytes, myoglobinuria, raised creatinine phosphokinase, LDH and transaminases, raised serum phosphate and potassium, and initially low serum calcium.

5 The chest symptoms may still be due to DVT. The tests are highly sensitive and specific for proximal vein thrombosis in symptomatic patients, but may miss small proximal and calf vein thrombi, which may grow and embolize later. Therefore a negative scan should be no deterrent to starting anticoagulants or requesting a ventilation/perfusion scan.

6 10%.

7 Colour venous duplex scanning.

8 a Doppler ultrasound ankle systolic blood pressure for arterial disease and venous duplex scanning for venous disease.
  b 57%.
  c 14%.

9 True – although manufacturers usually recommend a detector tuned to a higher frequency.

## Management

1 Repeated leg movement, raising the foot of the bed, and compression in an elastic stocking.

2 a True.

b False.

3   a  About 60%.

    b  About 30%.

4  False – the risk of haemorrhage from anticoagulants exceeds that of pulmonary embolism from factor V Leiden.

5  Elastic multilayer bandaging appears to be better than inelastic compression. Intermittent pneumatic compression adds to the effect of compression stockings.

6   a  20 weeks.

    b  43 weeks.

7   a  Ligation of perforating veins, which can now be performed with minimal scarring using endoscopic surgery.

    b  Povidone iodine, acetic acid and sodium hypochlorite probably help, although they are injurious to fibroblasts *in vitro.*

    c  Split skin grafts and excision and flap coverage.

8   a  A 36% reduction in ulcer size at 6 weeks, compared to 3% in the control group.

    b  Reduced leucocyte adhesion, increased red cell flexibility and increased formation of collagen and capillaries.